The Manuɛ

AAC

ASSESSMENT

Titles in the **Speechmark Editions** series:

The Manual of

AAC

ASSESSMENT

Arlene McCurtin &
Geraldine Murray

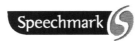

Many thanks
to Muireann McCleary
for comments and suggestions

Published by
Speechmark Publishing Ltd, Telford Road, Bicester, Oxon OX26 4LQ, United Kingdom
www.speechmark.net

002-3928/Printed in the United Kingdom/1010

British Library Cataloguing in Publication Data

McCurtin, Arlene
    The manual of AAC assessment
    1. People with disabilities – Means of communication 2. People with disabilities – Means of communication – Evaluation 3. Communication devices for people with disabilities
    4. Communication devices for people with disabilities – Evaluation
    I. Title II. Murray, Geraldine
    616.8'55'03

ISBN 0 86388 490 3
(Previously published by Winslow Press Ltd under ISBN 0 86388 200 5)

For

Dierdre, Ciaran and Ronan

About the Authors

Arlene McCurtin graduated as a speech & language therapist in 1985 and obtained her MSc in 1994. Currently head of the Speech & Language Therapy Department at the Central Remedial Clinic in Dublin, she has previously worked in both England and Canada. Her special interests are in feeding and AAC; she is the author of *The Manual of Paediatric Feeding Practice* (Speechmark Publishing, 1997).

Geraldine Murray is an occupational therapist and completed her undergraduate degree in 1979. She is currently head of the Occupational Therapy Department at the Central Remedial Clinic, Dublin, and is also an external lecturer for Trinity College, Dublin. She has previously worked in the United States as an Associate Assistant Professor in the Rehabilitative Sciences, Oklahoma University.

A core focus of both departments is the provision of augmentative and alternative communication assessment and therapy services.

Contents

Tables

Figures

Sample Forms

Preface

A picture paints a thousand words.

The intention of this manual is to provide practical guidelines to clinicians for understanding and conducting assessments of augmentative and alternative communication (AAC). It is particularly of relevance to the field of congenital paediatric disability as this is the area of work of the authors, but it is hoped that clinicians working in other areas of augmentative and alternative communication will be able to apply the information contained in this manual to their own field.

Furthermore, this book acknowledges that speech & language therapists and occupational therapists working in the field of augmentative and alternative communication may not have access to a range of specialised technological equipment that is ideally standard for carrying out assessments in this area. With this in mind, references are made to the utilisation of common everyday materials, where appropriate, to facilitate the assessment process.

In this manual the term augmentative and alternative communication (AAC) is used to refer to both low-tech (eg, communication boards) and high-tech (eg, communication aids) materials. Signing is not included in this definition for the purposes of this book, as the authors do not frequently use this mode in their professional work.

Knowledge of all the areas outlined in this manual is essential for the clinician working in the area of augmentative and alternative communication. For ease of understanding and to facilitate the assessment process, assessment areas have been segregated into chapters. However, the clinician should understand that assessment of augmentative and alternative communication is not about segregation of functions and areas, but rather an assimilation of knowledge of the abilities and needs of the individual across all domains.

Arlene McCurtin
Geraldine Murray
Dublin, June 2000

CHAPTER 1

Defining Augmentative and Alternative Communication

Introduction

Augmentative and alternative communication (AAC) involves the use of non-verbal means and systems to communicate. It is used to enhance an individual's communication skills, thereby facilitating communicative, social and personal development, and increase independence. AAC can be broadly classified into three groups: no technology, low-technology and high-technology.

No-tech means include:
- Natural gestures
- Eye signals
- Facial expression
- Sign language

Low-tech systems do not typically involve voice output. Examples are:
- Objects
- Tactile symbols
- Eye-transfer (E-Tran)/eye-gaze boards
- Rotary scanners
- Communication boards, wallets and books

High-tech systems are communication aids which typically produce digitised (recorded) or synthesised (artificial) voice, replicating the verbal mode, and are more typical of the way human beings communicate with each other (that is, speech). Examples are:

- Single channel voice output switches such as the Bigmack® switch. Although these switches produce voice, their function and range are significantly more limited than the more complex devices. Rumble & Larcher (1998) have classed these small static devices as 'light-tech'.
- Communication aids that come relatively unprogrammed such as the Macaw®, Alphatalker® and Chatbox®, and predominately rely on individuals to store words and phrases in them. These typically use recorded (digitised) speech.
- Communication aids with software that are either language programmes or can facilitate development of a language system. These typically use synthetic speech. Examples of these are the Deltatalker® and the Dynavox®. These can be either dedicated or integrated devices.
- Hardware, such as personal computers or laptops, onto which communication or language software can be loaded and used as a communication aid. Software such as the literacy based EZKeys® package can be used in this way.

High-tech systems can be further classified as follows:

1 Single Displays (Static) versus Multiple Displays (Dynamic).
   - *Static* devices typically have an unchanging overlay and in this way are like communication boards. The range of words and phrases stored on these devices can be significantly enlarged by combining icons (symbols) to form new communication messages. Typical examples of this type of aid are Liberator®, Macaw®, Eclipse® and Spokesman®.
   - *Dynamic* devices more closely resemble communication books in that the communication messages are stored in pages or files and the user can turn from page to page. They more closely resemble traditional computers and are called dynamic because the screen

is not static. Typical of this type of aid are the Dynamite®, Vanguard® and Cameleon®.

2   Dedicated versus Integrated.
  ◆ *Dedicated* devices have only one purpose – that of a communication aid. Communication aids are generally becoming less dedicated over time however, as facilities are being added as standard to them. These include environmental controls (for example, for operating the television). Their primary purpose remains communication and they can still be classed as dedicated. An example of a dedicated static aid is a Deltatalker®. An example of a dedicated dynamic aid is a Dynamite®.
  ◆ *Integrated* devices function as communication aids but are not primarily communication aids; they have multiple uses. The hardware involved provides other functions such as environmental controls and word-processing facilities. An example of a dynamic integrated aid is the Cameleon®.

Terminology

The term 'augmentative and alternative communication' (AAC) is used in this manual because it is familiar and recognisable. However, it is our belief that implementation of an AAC system should not be viewed as an *alternative* to speech, that is, a replacement of a person's current communication system. Instead it should be constructed as complementary. Experience tells us that every person who requires AAC intervention is already a communicator, albeit perhaps in a less formalised and less easily understood manner by the global community. Communication is already established through potentially a number of modes. These may include:

• Behavioural communication (eg, crying)
• Gross physical movements (eg, turning away)
• Non-verbal signals (eg, eye movements for 'yes' and 'no')
• 'Unintelligible' speech

Therefore, one of the functions of AAC implementation is to establish rapport with these modes rather than to replace them.

The Questions of AAC

Why Assess for AAC?
AAC assessments are carried out for a number of reasons.

- To speak or not to speak? When given this option the vast majority of us elect to have the ability to speak. Unfortunately, some people are not born with the potential to produce verbal language, perhaps due to a physical disability. In today's world, we increasingly have the ability to facilitate these individuals by providing them with a means of communicating through either low-tech or high-tech methods. For those of us who have seen the rapid transformation of both children and adults who are introduced to AAC, the question of 'Why?' does not exist. Providing people who are communication impaired with a means of expressing their thoughts, feelings, needs and desires is sufficient reason.
- Communication involves a minimum of two people. When we ask 'Why AAC?' we must answer with reference to this concept. For if communication involves two people and one of them cannot communicate as effectively as his potential dictates, then we cannot label the interchanges that occur as communication as we know it.
- It has often been said that communication-impaired people have a right to communicate. We would strongly agree with this. That right becomes important if it is claimed by a person through a desire to communicate using AAC, in addition to an interest in communicating and in developing their communication repertoire.
- AAC can achieve several vital goals.
  - It allows a person to express his personality/individuality.
  - It allows a person control over his environment.
  - It facilitates connection with people.
  - It contributes to that person's potential for independence.
  - It demands the respect for that person that is due him as an individual.

    The use of an AAC device puts the onus on a communication partner to construct the user more positively and more equally. We have found that some listeners have had to re-adjust their attitude and re-evaluate the person they thought they knew. This is most evident with adult users newly introduced to AAC who can now exert some control over situations. This probably upsets a balance long established where the communication partner has typically maintained control and dominated the interaction – in other words, communicated *at,* and not *with.*

The implementation of AAC does not necessarily resolve problems of interaction and any AAC prescription needs to be accompanied by intensive training of both user and carers. In other words AAC implementation is not a miracle cure; it is a part-solution to the bigger problem of the overall disorder such as the physical disability.

Prior to any assessment, the team must determine the purpose of that assessment. Two particular questions that should be asked are:

1   To what extent should the system function communicatively for the individual?
     Total use – to substitute for verbal output
     Partial use – to be used only in certain situations.

     An adult for whom we carried out an assessment was severely unintelligible to unfamiliar listeners including the assessment team. She was readily intelligible to family and friends however, and was quite sure that she needed something portable and small in message content with a set number of stored phrases. This was to be used only for certain situations, and after demonstration of the available range she made an easy choice to suit her own individual needs.

2   Should the device be dedicated or integrated?
     Do the individual's needs involve communication alone?
     Are the individual's needs more general, including other issues such as word processing?

When to Assess for AAC?

The assessment of an individual for AAC would be appropriate in the following circumstances:

- When an individual's communication needs cannot be met by his current communication modes/system.
- When the individual is capable of using AAC cognitively and receptively relative to his expressive ability – that is, the person's potential to communicate is impacted upon by his disability. This reference to cognitive functioning does not necessarily imply that a person's cognitive functioning needs to be in line with his chronological age.
- When an individual's ability to express himself intelligibly is limited to a few familiar communication partners, and it is desirable or necessary for him to expand his range of communication partners and communication skills.
- When people in an individual's environment are unwilling or unable to understand that individual's communications and consequently the communication-impaired person desires an improvement in his communication ability.
- When oral motor therapy input has been unsuccessful in producing positive change, or is deemed not to make sufficient improvement, if implemented.
- When the individual has a desire to use AAC and realises his potential in that area.
- When the individual is not satisfied with the limitations of his communication skills.
- When communication needs have changed because of changes in that individual's life (for example, moving school), or because he have outgrown his current system.

AAC assessment should take place as soon as is possible. The idea that an individual is too young or not ready for AAC is outdated, along with the notion of prerequisites. AAC systems can be utilised to train skills not already present. Reasons for this include, firstly, that a person can be trained either to associate communication symbols with intentional communication, or to switch and scan, and secondly good models of communication should be in place before maladaptive styles develop which can significantly hinder the implementation of AAC at a later stage.

Where to Assess for AAC?
Assessment for AAC prescription is incomplete if carried out only in the isolation of a clinic room. Assessment should take place:

1   In the clinic for specific activities. The use of a quiet, non-distracting environment can result in an improved idea of a person's potential. One individual we assessed was extremely distracted by auditory (eg, a person talking) and visual (eg, a person passing his wheelchair) stimuli resulting in continuous asymmetrical tonic neck reflex (ATNR) movements, and significantly affecting the accurate use of a switch to select messages. In the contained environment of a clinic room, he was able to demonstrate an ability to access and scan far superior to that demonstrated previously.

2   In the everyday environment of the individual and in commonly occurring situations. This is particularly true in the pre- and post-trial periods of assessment. AAC prescription will not necessarily work unless the clinician is fully aware of:
   • The individual's communication needs within those everyday environments.
   • The individual's ability to use an AAC system within those environments.
   • The support systems available in those environments.

Whom to Assess for AAC?
Communication aids are used to provide a system of communication to an individual whose ability to communicate and level of communication are not refined or formal enough to ensure successful communication. These are individuals who are unable to produce speech, perhaps due to a disability such as a physical handicap which affects oral motor function.

However, some candidates for augmented communication may produce some speech, but their ability to communicate their messages is limited by poor intelligibility.

Candidates who present for AAC are usually classified into three main groupings: congenital, progressive and acquired disorders (see Table 1.1).

Table 1.1 *Candidates for AAC*

Congenital	Progressive	Acquired
Motor disorders eg, cerebral palsy, dyspraxia	Retts syndrome	Traumatic brain injury
	Leucodystrophies	Elective mutism
	Multiple sclerosis	CVA
Learning disability	Motor neurone disease	Post-surgery eg, laryngectomy
Sensory impairments		
Multiple and profound disabilities		

In summary, we can assess the following individuals:

1   Anybody whose potential to express themselves communicatively is impacted upon by their disability.
2   Anybody who expresses a desire for AAC and the motivation to use an AAC system.
3   Anybody who has the support systems available for implementing AAC, whether this is the individual himself or carers or locally based professionals.

As Shane (1986, p40) states:

> It is not possible to have generalised candidacy requirements for augmentative intervention because each intervention must be individualised.

Assessment Principles

There are a number of principles that can be applied to AAC assessments.

Multiple Modes Contribute to Successful Communication
Musselwhite & St Louis (1988) have written of AAC as a continuum:

Augmentative communication ⟶ Vocal speech

and discuss AAC in relation to output versus input. We think of communication modes as complementary and see the various modes of communication as interacting and dynamic. A number of researchers (for example, Beukelman & Mirenda, 1992) have discussed the *total* communication of the AAC user. We feel that when prescribing and implementing AAC, the individual must be acknowledged as a global communicator, and current communication modes should be documented and recognised. Therefore, in order to highlight the total communicator, communication with regard to an AAC user can be considered under the following headings:

a   Style and level of non-verbal communication
b   Style and level of vocal communication
c   Style and level of verbal communication
d   Style and level of augmentative and alternative communication

Continuous Assessment is the Standard
The medical model, which can be outlined as:

Assessment ⟶ Diagnosis ⟶ Treatment

has reduced relevance in AAC prescription as it cannot be seen as a one-stop process. AAC prescription tends to fall more into line with the concept of diagnostic assessment, with therapeutic input and training being seen as part of the prescription process. This model can be envisaged along the following lines:

Assessment → Training → Diagnostic therapy →
Re-assessment → Prescription

9

A clinician will rarely meet an individual needing AAC whose AAC requirements are immediately transparent. Even when this happens, it is our policy to consider the rental of a communication aid prior to its prescription. The reasons for this are:

a   The range of communication aids available
b   The individual's specific needs
c   Specific individual issues such as scanning
d   The need to establish motivational levels
e   The need to familiarise the individual, carers and professionals with the aid
f   The need to train individuals, carers and professionals in the communication aid
g   The need to increase the awareness of the individual, carers and professionals of the practical everyday issues of augmented communication generally.

It is only through an understanding of the everyday issues surrounding the use of a communication aid, that individuality can be recognised and addressed. Therefore the ideal model in our view works something like that described in Figure 1.1.

Technology Should not be Viewed as Primary in the Assessment Process
The individual is at the core of AAC prescription and implementation and it is the individual and not the technology who determines the way forward. It is very easy today to get carried away with the advances in technology and therefore to focus on this aspect. We need to remember that it is the individual's needs and abilities which guide the AAC prescription process. Once we do this, we can succeed in our efforts to utilise our skills and the technology to the best advantage. It is only when technology meets the needs of the individual that it can be said to be of use.

Speech, which is unique to humans, is now coming of age through both low and high technology for non-verbal individuals. Through AAC, we in the field are not just able to help individuals find a voice, but most importantly we are helping them to discover their uniqueness.

1 Receipt of referral

2 Contact with primary carers and professionals responsible for implementation

3 Retrieval of specific information from referral and local sources

4 Establishment of core person (contact) responsible for coordination

5 Pre-assessment observations by the speech & language therapist in the individual's everyday environments and for everyday situations

6 Completion by relevant people of pre-assessment questionnaires to establish communication modes, success and style

7 Completion of biographical questionnaire by immediate carers to establish case history, interests, etc

8 Evaluation 1 to include information session on AAC generally, AAC options, and commencement of assessment process

9 Evaluation 2/3

10 Advice on rental for diagnostic period

11 Training of individual and primary carers and professionals

12 Review and re-assessment

13 Advice on rental 2 if necessary

14 Further training for rental 2

15 Review

16 Prescription

17 Training

18 Ongoing contact with the core person

19 Review 1/2/3

Figure 1.1 *A proposed model of AAC assessment*

Funding does not Determine Prescription
The availability of funding does not determine whether the assessment will occur and what ultimately will be prescribed. While funding is integral to the eventual success of the project, the unavailability of funding should not inhibit a prescription being made.

AAC Implementation is not Based on the Notion of Prerequisites
As Reichle (1991) states:

> There is no conclusive evidence to support the premise that certain cognitive behaviours must be in place before an initial repertoire of communicative behaviour can be implemented.

The theory of cognitive or linguistic prerequisites for AAC, while helpful, is not mandatory for successful use of AAC. In our work, if we determine that an individual is not capable of operating a refined AAC system, we may still prefer to implement an appropriate system (eg, single-channel voice-output switch, tactile symbols) in a structured manner for the following reasons:

a The person can learn to *associate* using symbols with communication – that is, AAC is applied on a receptive rather than expressive basis initially.
b The person can associate symbols with positive feedback.
c The person can have experience of AAC.
d The person can experience successful communication.
e The new system may be used to substitute for or prevent maladaptive communication behaviours (eg, screaming) being used or developing.

We prefer to call this stage 'Pre-AAC'.

The Goal of Successful Prescription and Implementation is
Communicative Competence
Experience of successful communication and communicative competence are the goals of AAC implementation. With this in mind we must remember:

a   Multiple modes enhance the likelihood of success – for example, non-verbal signals + board + device.

b   Established modes that are intelligible and acceptable communicatively should be used in conjunction with AAC, for example, non-verbal 'Yes' and 'No' signals that are intelligible do not need to be replaced with voice output.

Prescription is not the Only Aim

The successful implementation of an AAC system does not only involve the actual prescription. It is a time-consuming process which should include:

Training of individuals, carers and professionals in:
+ The individual communication aid
+ AAC in general
+ Strategies for using the system successfully in the everyday environment
+ Switch use and scanning where appropriate
+ Problem solving

Development of the AAC system which may include:
+ How to add further symbols to a board
+ Storage of new pages on a communication folder or dynamic device
+ Development of the device alongside the ongoing development of the person

Adaptation to an individual's changing needs:
+ Upgrading an AAC system can involve the addition of elements such as environmental controls, link-up to a printer, or the prescription of a new device.
+ Downgrading an AAC system can happen if a person has a degenerative condition (eg, leucodystrophy) or has had a long and traumatic period of hospitalisation. One of our users 'forgot' the programme on his communication aid after a prolonged period in hospital and was no longer able to deal with the level of complexity he was accustomed to. A change, not in the communication aid but in the software, restored communication to him, although additional learning was involved.

- ◆ Access needs and switch control sites can change. We find this can especially happen after a growth spurt and can be difficult to rectify quickly if seating equipment cannot be prescribed fairly rapidly.
- ◆ Technology can become outdated and improved aids come on the market which meet a person's need more effectively. We typically find working with our population, that communication aids have a life span usually of between five to seven years.

Support Systems are Essential to Ensure Successful Implementation
Support systems of core people need to be identified in order to ensure successful implementation. It is not atypical for AAC systems to fail because their implementation has not been adequately and professionally supported. These support systems typically include the immediate carer and speech & language therapists. Providing training and assigning responsibility for the communication aid will go a long way to facilitating effective use of the AAC system.

Team Working is Essential to Ensure Successful Implementation
The team involved in AAC prescription is necessarily large due to the global nature of communication and its use in all environments, and the variety of factors affecting successful communication, for example, seating, physical condition, use of AAC systems in all situations.

There is a necessity however, for a few core people to lead and guide the process. We define the core team narrowly:

- The individual
- The speech & language therapist
- The occupational therapist (where there are issues around physical access to the aid)
- The carer

The consultative team can be extensive but is composed mainly of the following:

- Other carers
- Seating therapist

- Care staff
- Educational staff
- The company that supplies the product
- Technician

Pre-Assessment Results are Guide Posts
While the team should always ensure they have the results of linguistic, psychological, visual, auditory and other significant tests to hand prior to beginning the assessment, it should be remembered that:

Results from testing are only guidelines.

Our team tends to use standardised assessments, with adaptations so that people with physical disabilities can use them. However, we are very aware that standard tests are not standardised on the disabled population and as such are invalid, and many tests depend on motor responding which is difficult if not impossible for a large proportion of the physically disabled population.

With this in mind, we need to be aware that individuals who require AAC systems may not perform well on standardised testing (psychological or linguistic) because of the nature of their disability. We have found a tendency to underestimate a person's ability. Due to this sometimes gross underestimation, test results should be used as guidelines only, for example, to convey that a person has a basic vocabulary level. We know extremely competent communication aid users in their mid-twenties, who, while using the most complex software and linguistic productions, score at the equivalent of five-year-old levels on tests of language comprehension. Therefore, the idea is to utilise tests to tap potential.

Communication is Part of the Environment
AAC implementation is not going to be successful unless it is functionally set up and used in the environments and situations of the individual who has been recommended it. Therefore integration of the AAC system is vital. It should be remembered that communication does not occur in a vacuum.

CHAPTER 2

Indicators

Introduction

People often ask with regard to AAC:

> Who is appropriate for assessment and what levels do they need to attain prior to assessment?

We feel strongly that the somewhat uncompromising idea of prerequisites has reduced relevance in the field of AAC prescription. There is a significant number of the population who require AAC intervention who will need elements of practice and training, whatever level of AAC is being applied, prior to decisions about prescription being made. This reflects our opinion of AAC implementation as being a diagnostic type of input. With this in mind, the following guidelines around the issues of speech, language, literacy, physical and cognitive issues are discussed.

Speech Development

There are a number of indications of potential 'non-verbalness'. However, when addressing the AAC area, there are two general questions we must ask:

- Are there indications that the individual will not be able to use speech as a primary mode of communication?

- If the individual uses speech currently, is it significantly intelligible to support effective and successful communication?

In order to make it easier to answer the questions posed, we can class the individuals who attend for AAC assessment into groups. These groups are:

1   The potentially non-verbal individual
2   The confirmed non-verbal individual
3   The partially verbal individual

The Potentially Non-Verbal Individual
This is the very young child who chronologically is too young to be thought of as non-verbal. This child will not have had a history of failure of either the speech mode, or therapeutic input focusing on language and oral motor function.

We must therefore be aware of the potential for speech not developing as expected. This is particularly in light of the potential for development of maladaptive behaviours, and the need to provide a model of successful, concrete communication.

Therefore what factors must we consider when we meet this child? These can be grouped under two main headings: those relating to physical disability and those relating to oral motor function.

Physical disability
1   *The severity of the physical disability.* Generally, the more severe the handicap, the more likely a child is to require facilitation in all areas of his life. This includes mobility, independence and communication. For example, an individual with the quadriplegic (all four limbs affected) type of cerebral palsy is typically more involved than an individual with the diplegic (two limbs) type.
2   *The type of disability.* Cerebral palsy (CP) is a very broad term used to describe many types and levels of disability, each with its own variation. The child most at risk will have one of the more severe types such as the following:
   - CP with athetosis – muscle tone just below normal

- CP with choreoathetosis – muscle tone fluctuating from below to above normal
- CP with spasticity – muscle tone always above normal especially when in the moderate to high range
- CP with dystonic spasms – muscle tone fluctuating from below normal suddenly to high tone and then dropping down again just as quickly
- CP with ataxia – muscle tone a little low with poor coordination and occasional tremors
- CP with hypotonia – reduced muscle tone

The child who is born prematurely and some other young babies may not have a full diagnosis but some of the above signs will be evolving. The child may go on to develop cerebral palsy, or may be found to have an underlying metabolic disorder.

There are also young children with degenerative conditions such as Retts Syndrome or the leucodystrophies who lose the ability to speak. Typically, any individual with a condition which involves oral motor dysfunction must be seen to be at risk in terms of their speech development.

Oral motor functions
Please note that although the term '*oral*' is used in this context, reference is also made to pharyngeal and laryngeal functions.

1   *The degree of involvement of non-speech oral motor functions.* A child can demonstrate problems with oral motor functioning long before that child is expected to produce speech.

    a   The main evidence of potential problems are seen in the area of *feeding difficulties.* These can be evidenced for example by:
- Poor suck-swallow-breathe coordination
- Spillage of food
- Aspiration
- Inability to manage a range of consistencies
- Reduced endurance, and
- Gagging/choking

Not all children who have feeding problems go on to to be non-verbal.

b   *Sensory abnormalities* in the oral and facial areas may also be a factor. However, it must be pointed out that in our experience, children who present with sensory abnormalities in isolation, that is, not accompanied by oral motor dysfunction, are not at particular risk for the non-development of speech. Oral facial sensitivity problems can be evidenced as follows:
- Hyposensitivity or reduced sensitivity to touch
- Hypersensitivity or increased sensitivity to touch.

c   *Tonal problems* in the oral facial area, sometimes linked to overall tone problems in the body are classic indicators of potential oral motor dysfunction, and indeed the feeding difficulties noted above may result from problems in this area:
- Hypotonia or reduced muscle tone causing developments such as an open mouth posture and sluggish oral movements
- Hypertonia or increased tension of the muscles producing difficulties such as uncoordinated oral movements.

d   There are other *general indicators* of oral motor dysfunction which follow on from those noted above: for example, open mouth posture and significant drooling.

e   Another good indicator is evidence of *breathing problems* that is, breath support and control for speech production may not be sufficiently developed or developing. As speech production is dependent on controlled breath support, this will have obvious implications for speech development.

2   *The degree of involvement of speech oral motor functions.* This area can be classed into either reduced output or absence of output.

a   *Absence of vocal and/or verbal output.* Typically, young children follow a pattern of developmental milestones during their early years. Children whose production is so limited as to be classified as absent typically show no evidence of either vocal productions (vowels) or early verbal productions (that is, CV sequences such as 'ba', or CVCV sequences such as 'baba'). They can be rated as particularly severe if, for example:

- Vocalisations are not part of their spontaneous repertoire particularly as these develop initially on an unintentional basis.
- The child is generally very quiet.
- The parent finds it difficult to distinguish between early types of communication eg, a tired cry and a hungry cry.
- There is a lack of development of vocal and verbal imitation skills.

This pattern is typical of the child with a significant physical disability affecting the development and production of speech.

b *Reduction in the individual's output.* These children typically reach some early milestones and may produce some vocalisations or verbalisations but these are limited.

- Output can be reduced in frequency that is, some productions are evident but these are significantly less than one would expect from a child developing speech normally.
- The range of productions can be limited both vocally and particularly verbally. For example, a child may produce 'ah' or 'ma' reliably but shows no evidence of developing a range of productions. That is, the individual's outputs are isolated and not built upon.
- The sequential or multisyllabic nature of speech may not be evident. For example, a single CV combination (eg, 'ba') may be produced but combined CV sequences, such as 'baba', are less frequent or absent.
- Those productions that do occur may not be produced as spontaneously as expected in normally developing children, requiring more effort and concentration particularly when meaning is attached to them.

We would use these indications to guide us towards implementing an early AAC system. In essence, waiting for speech to emerge carries more risk than implementing AAC and facilitating perhaps speech development and certainly AAC development.

The Confirmed Non-Verbal Individual
This group is the easiest to recognise and therefore determine AAC suitability for as they are obviously non-verbal.

1   They present as non-speaking at an age at which all or most developmental milestones should have been achieved and are patently not acquired. This group is more visible the older they become.
2   They may have had a long (sometimes prolonged) history of therapeutic input focusing on oral motor production and have remained effectively non-verbal.
3   They may have had a low-tech (eg, communication board) communication system implemented. This is not always the case however, even with relatively old individuals (old by AAC implementation standards). We still meet teenagers and adults who have had no history of AAC implementation but who are very obvious candidates for an AAC system.
4   They may have developed strategies (eg, pointing) for improving intelligibility or facilitating understanding of their output.

The Partially Verbal Individual
Partially verbal individuals are readily identifiable by the following:

1   The use of speech as the primary communication mode.
2   In some cases there is a history of unsuccessful speech production therapy and AAC implementation.
3   The transparent unintelligibility of their speech to unfamiliar people and their ineffective use of speech with these communication partners.
4   Their reported intelligibility to familiar communication partners and their reportedly effective use of speech with these partners. However, after probing in depth, the speech & language therapist usually finds that the range of 'intelligible' utterances is reduced generally, and

intelligibility is facilitated by contextual cues with these familiar communication partners. These individuals may not be good communicators in the areas of initiation and spontaneity.

5   The use of strategies to facilitate intelligibility. These include:
  ◆ Use of one-word utterances versus multi-word utterances
  ◆ Use of pictures or symbols in the environment
  ◆ Use of natural gestures or signing to support speech output
  ◆ Reliance on familiar partners to interpret for them
  ◆ Use of situational cues. For example, when such an individual is in a shop and he is buying a treat, the potential message range is limited and so interpretation is easier.

It must be noted that the judgement of intelligibility may not be as straightforward as it first appears and Dowden (1997) has called intelligibility 'a complex phenomenon'. Both Dowden (1997) and Kent *et al* (1994) have suggested rightly that we should consider a number of variables. General guidelines that can be used to assess the impact of this intelligibility are:

- Does articulatory and phonological assessment across situations (eg, school, home) indicate a problem?
- Does articulatory and phonological assessment across all levels of production (eg, single word, spontaneous speech) indicate a problem?
- Does the trained ear of the speech & language therapist have difficulty understanding the individual in spontaneous speech and without many contextual cues?
- Does the trained ear of the speech & language therapist have difficulty interpreting the speech of the individual with contextual cues, with repetition and during short productions?
- Has the individual a history of therapeutic intervention focusing on speech production which has been unsuccessful in producing significant change?
- Does the parent/carer/individual feel that the individual's communications are limited to certain people and situations?

If intelligibility is deemed to be a problem sufficient to warrant AAC implementation the following questions should then be asked:

- How does the individual construct his speech and rate the success of his communication attempts? Does his unintelligibility have a negative or motivating impact upon him?
- Does the individual want to augment his speech using AAC?
- How reliable is speech and how much should it continue to be used either as the primary mode or otherwise?
- Does the individual have the internal motivation to use AAC or are his needs fairly well met by speech and perhaps the limited number of communication opportunities available to him?
- Are the primary carers happy with speech as the sole mode of communication?
- Is the speech & language therapist happy with speech as the sole mode of communication?
- Would the support be available locally to implement an AAC system?

Please note that if internal motivation and external support are missing, so is a key to success. One may find the partially verbal individual unmotivated until a change in life occurs which presents new challenges, and perhaps difficult situations for him.

Language Levels

Standardised Testing
Language comprehension equivalent to the chronological age of the individual is a valuable asset, but it is not an essential ingredient for successful AAC use. The standard typically applied to individuals attending for AAC assessment is that there should be a gap between the levels of language comprehension and language expression in favour of the former. We feel that language comprehension levels should be used as a guideline only, given the very real difficulties of assessing these skills in the physically disabled population. Although we utilise standardised tests, we tend to rely more heavily on the results of our own criterion-referenced measures for leading the assessment process. This is due to the intrinsically more valuable information yielded by criterion-referenced tasks, and the difficulties inherent in using standardised instruments for individuals with physical disability. These difficulties arise due to the following factors:

- These instruments are not standardised on the population with physical disability and are therefore invalid.
- Most tests depend on some form of motor responding which is less possible because of the nature of physical disability.
- The individual's relative lack of world and communication experiences means that we find there are significant gaps in their linguistic skills which do not reflect effectively their potential.

These points reflect the vital difference in assessing the skills of this population. That is, that the clinician should be evaluating the individual's *potential to communicate* rather than basing recommendations solely on his ability as evidenced by linguistic, psychological or medical findings. These instruments should be used in conjunction with other results gained from the assessment process. This is one of the reasons why diagnostic therapy, criterion-referenced tasks and evaluation of all skills areas are vital. The experience and skills of this group tend to be limited because of the confines placed upon them by their disability. The clinician therefore should be giving individuals who attend for AAC assessment the opportunity to demonstrate their skills.

Therefore, in utilising standardised tests, the clinician should be aware of the limitations of these and should consider modifications to:

- Materials – for example, the enlargement of picture stimuli to facilitate a motor response or the use of eye signals.
- Procedures – for example, eliminating the motor response and using other forms of access such as row–column scanning.

Results can be interpreted using the standardised instruments but should be treated with caution for the following reasons:

- Modifications to procedures or materials may have been made thereby effectively invalidating the results.
- Tests are not standardised on the disabled populations.
- Consideration should be given to the reduced communication experience of individuals.

Criterion-Referenced Testing

Criterion-referenced tasks do not use standardised data. They are individual tasks which pertain only to the performance of the individual. Criterion-referenced tasks provide very individualised rather than generalised results. With this type of assessment, the clinician is basically asking the question:

Can the individual do this very specific task?

An example of this could be:

Can the person point to a picture on the upper left corner on a display using 32 pictures in total?

This assessment style provides information which is individual specific and therefore immediately usable. Criterion referenced tasks provide the clinician with absolutely relevant information relative to the specific goals of the assessment.

In unpublished research, McCurtin (1994) found that a significant proportion of therapists demonstrated a preference for the use of criterion-referenced measures for individuals presenting with a disability. Given our commitment to the early AAC group, criterion-referenced assessments have an extra value, as this is the group which typically is seen as 'untestable' and using these types of measures provides us with specific information which previously would not have been attainable.

In summary, formal assessment results should be used as guidelines only with criterion-referenced results providing the more specific and relevant information necessary for decision making regarding AAC. Mastery of skills is not essential given:

- Individuals have a right to consider AAC as an option, communication and independence being vital skills for them.
- We may not truly understand a person's potential until we implement diagnostic measures.
- We must rule out the possibility of maladaptive behaviours developing in lieu of the more refined communication skills.

Literacy

With individuals who have the potential to use writing and spelling as a means of communication this is obviously the preferable route for the following reasons:

- A literacy-based system can give the impression of a more able communicator who will therefore demand more respect and attention from communication partners.
- Literacy is a further refinement on picture-based systems.
- It will also give the person potential for use of word-processing systems, access to computers, printers and systems such as the Internet and e-mail.
- Individuals who can communicate using literacy skills are less restricted and have the potential to produce more unique communications than individuals whose systems are picture based.

The guidelines for assessing literacy skills and the problems associated with them are the same as for those of language assessment that is, problems with standardisation, modifications, etc. We tend to base our assessment of literacy skills on three areas:

1   Assessment results and informal knowledge from the professionals involved, for example, teacher, speech & language therapist.
2   Criterion-referenced measures based on literacy acquisition and vocabulary assessments for reading.
3   Ability to spell words, which is different from the ability to read. The ability to spell ensures greater and more effective use of a literacy system. It must be pointed out that spelling can be more difficult for this population, perhaps because of difficulties in practising and using spelling (especially if an AAC system is not implemented early on), and reduced ability to verbally rehearse sounds and words.

However, some literacy-based software now has the bonus of the *Prediction* feature for users. This is where the spelling of each letter in the sequence gives the user possible options so that full spelling of the word may not be required. This can greatly facilitate the use of literacy as a communication and word-processing tool in this population.

Physical Disability

When a person is being considered for an AAC assessment, their physical ability and disability must be evaluated by the physiotherapist and occupational therapist. Without speech the individual must use some other mode to signal communication. Normally the young baby initiates and responds by crying, smiling, eye gaze, and eventually touch and finger pointing, before using speech.

> The basis for producing these normal developmental skills is posture.

The main question to be asked in this context is:

> Does physical disability affect the development of motor control?

Motor control may be affected by physical disability. How much it is affected will depend on the severity and distribution of the impairment. The clinician should observe the abilities and changes caused by efforts to communicate.

Cognitive Issues

Prerequisites
The approach of relying on prerequisite skills to be established prior to implementing AAC options has been found by the authors to be unsatisfactory for the following reasons:

- As previously discussed, standardised assessments are often inappropriate when used with this population. On many occasions when individuals are referred for psychological assessment, the psychologists may report that IQ cannot be determined. We often find that:
  - Signals of communication are not being picked up.
  - There is a tendency to rely on verbal motor responses to test cognitive levels.

- ◆ There is a reluctance to utilise criterion-referenced procedures in favour of standardised instruments which can limit the individual being assessed.
- ◆ The communication signals are often misinterpreted.
- ◆ Communication opportunities and training in AAC systems (that is, a refined communication system) have been limited, both for the individual and the evaluator.

- Where a cognitive and/or language level is determined, this information is used in the process of assessment, as is the information obtained from other sources (eg, visual perceptual assessments). However, they do not provide the basis for an AAC system. This information may provide:
  - ◆ Starting points for assessment.
  - ◆ Guidelines for changing the AAC system either to increase or decrease the sophistication.

- Clinicians may spend many years waiting for skills to 'emerge' when they could be facilitating that very development important to communication in some individuals.

Different Systems Require Different Cognitive Abilities
It is true that different systems require different cognitive abilities and it is important for the clinician to understand these. For example:

- There is a progression in the recognition of symbols such as:
  - ◆ Objects
  - ◆ Photographs
  - ◆ Pictures
  - ◆ Line drawings

- Selection through scanning (indirect selection) is a more difficult task than pointing (direct selection).
- Making a choice between two pictures by eye pointing requires less cognitive ability than using an electronic device.

Effect of Skills Other than Cognition

It is also true that some individuals who have the cognitive ability to use a sophisticated system, such as a 128 overlay on a static device, are not able physically to cope with the demands of access through a switch. Therefore, physical functioning, and not cognition hinders the application of AAC or the individual's ability to demonstrate that cognitive ability. Physical and sensory skills can have a big impact on a person's performance during assessment, and their use of a communication system.

It is therefore important not to be restricted by cognitive prerequisites or reliance on cognitive testing. The clinician should look to:

- Establishing motivation to communicate
- Assessing means of communication
- Promoting communication by all partners in all environments.

CHAPTER 3

Some Considerations Prior to AAC Assessment

Introduction

Both the ability of the individual and the characteristics of the AAC systems must be borne in mind during the assessment process. To understand AAC systems, we must first look at the general features which run through most systems. This will facilitate an understanding of why specific areas are targeted during the assessment process. This chapter outlines a number of important areas and of their implications for assessing the individual for AAC.

Prior to assessment, the clinician should ask:

- Does the individual have an AAC system already?
- If so, has this system been used successfully?
- If so, what are the specific characteristics of the system in particular in terms of the:
  - ◆ language
  - ◆ literacy
  - ◆ symbols
  - ◆ integration
  - ◆ access
  - ◆ scanning
  that have been successfully utilised?

- Are there features which have not been successfully utilised and if so, why not?
- Both extrinsic and intrinsic factors are important to successful communication. Intrinsic factors, such as physical abilities, sensory skills and cognitive levels are vital in determining appropriate prescription. However, factors extrinsic to the individual, such as the input received, motivators for the individual and carer interaction, also determine the potential for successful implementation.

Interaction

Often, in evaluating the potential of an individual for an AAC system, we neglect the interactional processes which can both facilitate and hinder the prescription process and the successful outcome of AAC. To ensure both that a prescription is appropriate and the outcome successful, it may also be important to observe and evaluate the interaction between the individual and the primary carer. This will be particularly helpful in the following ways:

- *To identify whether the carer is responding to the individual's signals*. If not, there will be implications for both the development of communicative intent and reduced frequency of successful communication experiences. This will serve to frustrate the individual and potentially reduce the level or presence of communication intent.
- *Identify the communication 'bond' between carer and individual*. This may help in deciding on the implementation of an AAC system. Reduced communication 'pickup' between carer and individual may mean preliminary work on interaction is necessary prior to prescribing an AAC system.
- *Identify the individual who carries the burden of communication* – that is, the most communication weight. Shared communication offers the greatest potential for successful AAC implementation.

Cognitive Issues

What cognitive issues are involved in AAC? At its simplest level we are looking for a reaction to stimuli, from which we can attempt to establish the motivation to communicate. The following are some of the cognitive processes utilised in AAC.

Attention and Listening Skills

To communicate with someone, one has to be able to gain and hold the attention of a person, at the most basic level. Greater attention skills are required to learn the meaning of symbols, commit them to memory, and use them to communicate. Listening skills are also important for interaction. They are particularly vital for individuals who have little or no vision.

Cause and Effect

This is an early stage in development. The child learns that there is a direct reaction/response to an action. For example, press a switch and a tape recorder plays a song. Understanding this concept is vital for an individual both in terms of access and communication.

Turn Taking

Communication is an interactive process. All communication partners need to learn to take and wait their turn. This is particularly relevant to AAC where the verbal partner too often dominates the interaction, and where the delay in responding by the non-verbal individual often destroys natural turn-taking rules. Gestures used to communicate needs and wants may be ignored. The individual may learn to be passive and not to initiate or continue conversation.

Memory

Memory skills are utilised for visual, auditory and motor learning. At the basic level the individual must remember the object in order to learn object permanence. At communication aid level, the memory load is greater. For example, when utilising semantic compaction on a static device or combining symbols on a symbol system such as Bliss®, each icon or symbol can have a different meaning depending on the combination with which it is used. For example:

Name + Sun = Sun

or

Rainbow + Sun = Yellow

Individuals with poor attention skills can work only for short periods on new activities. They require repetition of new and learned material in order to commit them to long-term memory.

Problem Solving
At the early stages of development, problem solving may be achieved in a random manner, by trial and error, for example, trying to put a square peg into a round hole and eventually trying the round hole. Children do learn to problem solve by experience, but also by observation. As the child matures, the ability to problem solve should become more sophisticated. The child can understand different approaches to the problem and use reasoning process to solve new challenges.

Decision Making
A voluntary response requires a decision to be made. The process of communication requires decision-making abilities at different levels depending on the sophistication of the interaction. The use of a communication aid requires decision-making ability, remembering the correct sequence of icons and/or pages, and deciding on using them. Problem-solving and decision-making skills become more demanding as the person's need and ability to communicate grows, and the complexity of the communication system increases.

Visual Perception
Visual perception is the interpretation of what we see. It is a developmental process, which can continue into the teenage years. There are many assessments available to the clinician to assess visual perception on its own, and also visual motor perception/interpretation.

Visual motor integration is the process of performing a visual motor act, for example, copying a block design in 3D. If an individual copies the design incorrectly, knows that it is incorrect but cannot correct it, the problem is of a visual motor nature. If the design is copied incorrectly, but the individual perceives it to be correct then it is a visual perceptual problem.

Normal visual perceptual ability allows us to identify shapes (for example, between ♥ and □), distinguish between subtle differences (for example, between the letters *d* and *b*), recognise such things as pictures, line drawings and letters, in different sizes, styles and colours. It allows us to focus on the relevant picture, from among others. When objects or pictures are presented to an individual, the type of background, spacing, layout, size and number will vary according to his stage of visual perceptual development.

When an individual has difficulties with visual perception, too many stimuli are visually confusing and the individual cannot concentrate on the task. Four pictures on the four corners of an E-tran frame may be all that some individuals can cope with. It is helpful in the early stages to present objects, pictures etc, in a left-to-right, top-to-bottom format as most voice-output device displays and written materials are presented in this way.

When visual perceptual difficulties are identified, steps must be taken to allow for these difficulties when presenting materials to the individual. Visual perceptual training programmes must be instigated along with regular re-evaluation of abilities. This will facilitate the upgrading of the AAC system.

Motor Planning and Motor Control
This is an important area for the individual, so that a voluntary action can be carried out and repeated. This requires the following abilities:

- To make a movement
- To receive sensory feedback
- To interpret that feedback
- To refine and plan the next movement so that the motor control becomes automatic and requires little conscious effort.

If the individual has difficulties with motor planning every sequence of movement is experienced as new. When learning to touch type, it is very difficult to persuade oneself not to look at the keys and one's fingers appear to have a mind of their own, hitting unwanted keys. Over time however, the movements become more refined, less awkward, require less effort and the motor control seems easy.

Motor planning and control can be very difficult to achieve when a person has a physical disability. It is made more difficult if there is also a learning disability.

Sequencing of Tasks

Having waited one's turn, to then use a switch or direct access requires a large amount of task sequencing. For many people the waiting time can be very difficult as they anticipate the right moment to hit the switch without acting too early or too late.

Sequencing has further relevance to AAC systems. The individual who is able to use a number of symbols/icons to construct words and sentences will have the potential for more developed communication than the individual who cannot.

Communication and Language Features

The more developed an individual's linguistic ability, the greater the chances for the individual using a more linguistically complicated AAC system, which can in turn serve to help him in communicating most of his needs. Language issues need to be considered on a number of levels.

Functions

Language is useful only if it is communicated by the individual. It is therefore essential in AAC that prescription is targeted at individuals who demonstrate a need and desire to use communication (although at the severest levels of disability, association work can facilitate this development). Examples of functions to be assessed include:

- Shared attention
- Turn taking
- Communicative intent
- Early language signals, such as confirmation and negation, etc.

These are vital language skills. Clearly, language functions can be an important indicator of the potential of the individual to benefit from AAC intervention.

Vocabulary

An individual's vocabulary skills will affect his ability to utilise and benefit from AAC prescription. It also serves to facilitate understanding of which level and type of AAC systems are appropriate for that individual.

The questions that must be asked are as follows:

1   *What is the level of the individual's vocabulary development currently?*
    This will help to determine the current AAC needs. For example, can
    the individual understand vocabulary only at noun level, or is more
    complex vocabulary such as verbs, adjectives and pronouns a
    receptive skill? Deciding on an AAC system whether high- or low-tech
    in nature, and implementing it will need to take account of this. If
    nouns are the level of vocabulary development in an individual, then
    the symbols used should represent this. For example: the symbol
    Television would directly relate to the word 'Television'.
        We do not necessarily mean that the language used with all
    symbols would be single word nouns in this case, as part of our
    intention is to incorporate other concerns for example, language
    development and social content. So the symbol *Television* in this case
    may be translated in voice-output devices as 'Turn the TV on'.
        The individual who has a limited vocabulary level may benefit
    from a less complicated device with a limited range of vocabulary
    and placing relatively limited demands on the user – for example,
    four, eight or sixteen symbols.

2   *What is the individual's potential for vocabulary development?*
    This will have relevance for the AAC system's capacity to grow with
    the individual and for its internal organisation.

Association and Categorisation Skills
An individual who has these skills will be able to understand how
individual items are organised and how they relate to each other; as a
result he will have the potential to use more complex communication
systems. Analysis of the individual's ability in this area can help in
deciding how to organise a low- or high-tech system, and whether static
or dynamic systems are more suited to the individual's cognitive style. For
example, the individual who demonstrates good categorisation ability
will be able to utilise a *category-based* system (whether low- or high-tech).
An individual who demonstrates good association skills will be able to use
a device which employs *semantic compaction* rules.

- *Categorisation.* Category-based systems function by storing vocabulary on pages, organised according to categories. Examples of these are the Food Page, School Page, Places Page, etc.
- *Semantic compaction.* Semantic compaction is an encoding technique which involves the ability to combine elements to form new constructions or meanings. For example, the symbol *apple* used in isolation will only refer to that object, a concrete association. However, when used in conjunction with another symbol, the meaning can change for example, *Apple + Hot* may mean 'Pie'. This is less transparent and involves an ability to understand that language and symbol combinations can produce meanings other than the obvious.

Musselwhite & St Louis (1988) have identified conditions under which words/icons are combined. The reason or way icons are combined to form new meanings varies. Some of these include:

a   *Categories* eg, all words from the same category will start with the same icon (such as *eye* representing body parts)
b   *Functions* eg, *Apple = eat*
c   *Character* (features) eg, *Sun = hot*

This feature can also involve the use of more abstract language abilities.

d   *Associations* (conventionalisms) eg, an elephant never forgets
e   *Other means* (multiple meanings) eg, *Eye = I.* Another example is the question starter on Language, Living and Learning® (LLL) software. This is *Witch,* the word sounding like the question 'Which?'

We typically find that individuals who demonstrate potential for this type of system do so quickly and naturally, although there are others who can be taught this skill. The benefit of this skill is the ability to create more communication messages from a relatively limited set of words and symbols.

We find this area a particularly important consideration as it appears that individuals may have style preferences which have significant implications for the system to be prescribed and implemented. It is our experience that identifying which, if any, of the two areas/styles – categorisation and semantic compaction – the individual demonstrates a preference for, will significantly facilitate the decision-making process. The individual preference appears to be related to cognitive style.

Some individuals perform equally well on both, but they often report a preference for one style over the other. Baker (1985) has pointed out why this may be – that is, that semantic compaction makes use of recognition memory, whereas category-based systems make use of recall memory. Therefore, cognitive style can be a predictor for the prescription of an AAC system.

It is not yet clearly understood how large a part recognition memory plays versus the individual's language skills when learning and using semantic compaction sequences. It is probably initially learned through association, and then recalled in use through recognition memory.

Grammatical and Syntactical Understanding
Is the individual able to combine language elements to form syntactic or morphological constructions? If the individual can use SVO (Subject + Verb + Object) constructions (eg, *David kicks ball)*, or understand tense markers to reflect tense appropriately, then the system implemented needs to reflect this ability to facilitate greater communication and cognitive abilities.

In order to combine words, the individual should have an understanding of sentence parts, although again, this is not essential to the use of a low- or high-tech system, as communication can be achieved in absence of syntax, and it can be taught along with general language and AAC development. However, an individual who is capable of utilising these structures to communicate has the capacity to produce more accurate messages and is less dependent on his communication partner.

Interestingly in Smith's (1996) research, she found non communication-impaired individuals who used AAC boards relied heavily on semantic and/or communication content rather than complete syntactical or grammatical structures. Furthermore, while we all understand that individuals may, due to time or listener constraints, need to produce attention-getting words which are heavy in semantic meaning rather than syntactic accuracy, there are many users who are capable of accurate syntactical or grammatical constructions and deserve the opportunity to be able to use them, should the need or desire arise.

The implications of this are of course that systems should be laid out to incorporate these skills and with regard to high-tech systems, the clinician should also be aware of the capacity of the system to incorporate or produce these constructions. Some software for example, Liberator® programmes such as LLL® and Unity®, have these inbuilt, as do some dynamic systems such as the Dynavox® range. Other systems may not have this capacity unless the information is programmed into it. To this end, prior to the assessment, the clinician is best to familiarise herself both with the range of devices on the market and the particular features of these devices.

Literacy

Some individuals will be able to read words and because of the flexibility of literacy as a communication tool for a non-verbal person (no system can be programmed with all possible utterances no matter how effectively designed), this needs to be considered in the evaluation process. However, most important in this is the assessment of the ability to spell – that is, to produce words, not merely to understand them in the written form. Therefore spelling needs to be assessed in the following ways:

1   Spelling of *common words.*
2   Ability to *part spell*. For example, if an individual can tell a communication partner what letter a word starts with, the range of possibilities is reduced, which facilitates interpretation. Additionally, some high-tech devices have encoding and prediction facilities which would make use of this skill. For example:
    • A single letter on a device such as the Lightwriter® can represent a phrase eg, *H* can be programmed to mean 'How are you?'.
    • Some programmes have predictions facilities in spelling programmes (eg, EZ Keys®) where if an individual can part spell, options will be produced. For example, an individual may want to spell the word 'Drink'. The spelling of the first letter will produce a variety of options of words starting with the letter D. If the second

letter is added to spell 'Dr' the list of options will be amended to include only words starting with 'Dr' and will possibly include the target word which the person can then select.

3   Ability to learn to spell *new words* for its obvious potential.

Symbols

When evaluating symbols, the clinician will need to consider a number of areas. Typically, the higher an individual's level within each area, the more complex the potential AAC system can be to most fully meet the needs of that individual. It is important to point out that an individual's abilities are not static and can change over time and therefore assessment in each area represents only current levels and current potential (at the time of testing).

Level of Representation
What symbolic level can an individual understand and use? Symbols can be evaluated in order of concreteness to abstractness (outside of system type). Hierarchical order follows developmental progression and is generally as follows:

1   Objects
2   Miniature objects (toys)
3   Photographs
4   Coloured pictures
5   Black-and-white line drawings
6   Abstract symbols and
7   Words.

In evaluating an individual's symbolic level, it is not essential to either follow the hierarchical progression or complete all levels. The clinician will usually understand what the individual is capable of achieving and work within that range. For example, a profoundly cognitively-impaired individual is unlikely to need literacy assessment and may not be able to understand photographs as symbolic representations. In this case evaluating objects should be sufficient. Similarly higher-level candidates may need evaluation only at line drawings and literacy levels.

Additionally, in programmes that accompany some high-tech devices, the symbol sets can be different to those used more commonly for both low- and high-tech systems. These include Dynasyms® used on the Dynavox® range, and Liberator® products, some of which programmes on the higher-level devices having more complex symbols than black-and-white line drawings and relying heavily on abstract or figurative associations. These are usually assessed by trialling the individual on a number of them directly (or copies of the device overlays). Some individuals will understand the more abstract symbols naturally; for others it may not be very relevant as they may utilise their memory to *learn* the location and meanings of symbols.

System Type

Although most centres who provide an AAC service tend to rely on one symbol system for reasons of clarity and familiarity, there are many symbol systems available for use. The predominant sets used are:

- Rebus®
- PCS® (Picture Communication Symbols), and
- Bliss®

Bliss® which had seen a major decline in use in recent years, has seemed to have experienced a renewal of interest. One of the reasons for this may be its facility for combining symbols to make parts of speech. However, it is less transparent than other systems which tend to be more immediately easily recognisable by users and communication partners. This immediacy has seen the growth in the use of these more transparent systems. It must be pointed out that the more abstract systems have a valuable use, and we have found users who have a prolonged history of Bliss® board use take easily to high-tech systems which use semantic compaction rules.

As noted previously, while the individual is at the core of the decision making, other factors such as systems already used in that individual's environment need also to be considered.

Size of Symbols

Again this will not necessarily apply to all candidates. The golden rule really is the smaller the symbol an individual is able to use, the greater the range of communication messages which can be stored on the AAC system. Some points need to be made with regard to this topic.

- The size of symbols has most relevance for individuals who use static devices or communication boards. These systems by the nature of their organisation are limited in their expansion capabilities.
- Some dynamic systems now have options which include symbol magnification and this may mean that the effect of symbol size will have reduced impact for certain individuals.
- Some individuals will need larger symbol sizes naturally, due to visual impairments or scanning difficulties.
- Sometimes the nature of the symbols will affect the range of options available for example, the use of objects.

Number of Symbols
Again, the greater the number of symbols on a system, the greater the range of communication messages generally available to the individual. There is no obvious benefit to being able to use a maximum number of symbols unless a static device is being considered, and unless this aspect is appropriate for the individual. It is the individual's abilities which will determine suitability of the various options. It is also the combination of skills which is vitally important.

For example, if an individual has the ability to select from 128 symbols but cannot semantically compact, then a system such as the device which employs semantic compaction cannot be of optimum use. However, if symbol size and number need to be reduced to accommodate the individual's particular needs, and a categorisational or dynamic system is appropriate, then this does not necessarily negatively impact on the user as multiple pages can be used on his system to accommodate this. However, it can make the system and the individual's use of it more laborious due to the fact that the individual has to go between multiple pages. It also has important implications for low-tech systems – for example, with regard to how a communication board should be arranged (how many symbols per block/page).

Combining Symbols

The issue of using symbols together has already been covered in the previous section when discussing organisation and style.

1   *Semantic compaction.* As discussed previously, this is a feature available on static devices such as Delta Talker® and Chatbox®. This type of encoding relies heavily on the individual's ability to remember associations but may be less based on recall than recognition. If an individual is capable of using this technique, the memory load can be enormous and a system grows more cumbersome as more semantic compaction options are used. Therefore, it is important for the clinician to ascertain the following: can the individual understand the concept of semantic compaction and can the individual remember a variety of semantic compaction messages?

2   *Use of single symbols on levels.* One symbol can mean a different message on each level. The Blackhawk® for example, has a maximum of 16 symbols on one level, and four levels. Pressing a level icon/button can move the individual to a different level, and thereby facilitate use of the same symbol for a different message. For example:
Level 1, Symbol 1 = 'Hello, my name is'
Level 2, Symbol 1 = 'I live in'
Level 3, Symbol 1 = 'I need to use this to communicate'
and so on.

3   *Use of locators/indicators* or symbols which add meaning to a symbol or extend the range of the message. For example with Bliss® an individual can locate the symbol *Happy* and then the symbol for *Opposite of* to communicate 'Sad'.

4   *Combining symbols to make syntactically and grammatically correct utterances.* These topics have been covered in the section on language. The ability to use syntactically and grammatically correct productions can produce more accurate messages and reduce dependency on the communication partner and guesswork.

Such information will help in the layout of the communication board or dynamic device, and on a high-level static system help in determining the programme to be chosen.

5   *Use of master/index pages* which function to direct the communication partner to vocabulary stored on category-based (eg, People, School, Equipment) pages.

6   *Other encoding techniques* which can range from simple to complex. An example is Alpha encoding, such as that seen on the Lightwriter® where a single letter when used in combination with a Memory button can produce a stored phrase. This is particularly valuable for often repeated information such as favourite food in a restaurant or identification information. An example is:

Memory key + H = 'Hello, how are you? My name is . . .'

Access
Access to AAC systems can be by direct selection or by indirect selection/ scanning.

Direct Access
This is achieved by touching or pointing directly to the desired choice (eg, object, picture), by using a body part, eg, fingers, eyes, toes or an assistive device such as a head pointer, track ball, light or optical pointers.

Direct access methods are generally faster than scanning and usually easier to understand. However, there are some drawbacks:

• The optical and light pointers can be difficult for young children to understand.
• They also require quite accurate targeting.
• Individuals may access large, well-spaced targets directly but are unable to continue with this method as the number of targets increases, and size and spacing decreases.

Scanning
There are basically three methods of scanning which are used in conjunction with a switch.

• *Automatic scanning*. The device controls automatic scanning and the individual operates a switch at the desired location.

- *Step scanning.* The movement of the cursor is controlled by the individual and chosen by stopping at the desired target or operating a second switch.
- *Inverse scanning.* Constant pressure is kept on the switch until the target is reached and then the switch is released.

These methods require different levels of motor control. Efficient and accurate switch control is necessary for all. To facilitate assessment and training the speed of scanning and the acceptance time for switch selection can be altered. The individual needs to be able to visually scan all the target locations so as to select the desired target.

Indirect Access by Switch
To develop independent functional use of a switch, there are a number of steps which may need to be worked on. Not every individual will require work or assistance on all stages.

- Some individuals with physical disabilities will understand immediately the effect of activating the switch, and will have sufficient motor control and effective positioning equipment to master the skill almost immediately. However most of the children and some of the adults we see have difficulty with both the understanding and the motor control. Assessment of switch use is a continuous process which may need to be completely readdressed a number of times.
- At the basic level understanding and achieving 'cause and effect' are the first independent skills. The individual must be motivated by the desire to make it happen, particularly if it requires overcoming physical difficulties. Most young children with physical disability do not gain such experiences by their own random movements. The opportunities for trials must be taken to the child.
- If the individual does not have a current supportive seating system, but requires one, this must also be addressed. Some individuals may be working on developing motor control for switch use through ongoing therapy. The child may be working while on the floor or supported by an adult while operating the switch. This can be a useful diagnostic period for finding the best method of access.

- At the same time a seating system may be being developed and regular trial periods will be necessary to evaluate how functional the seating system is. Some individuals with severe physical disabilities have great difficulty accommodating to seating systems which, in an effort to provide stability, reduce the individual's movements. This requires a lot of liaison among the therapists, parents, carers and the seating specialists.

Scanning

Visual Scanning
Visual scanning is a complex skill, which is made up of a number of components.

- *Motor.* The individual must have the motor control for aligning the head and body positions so that the eyes can be directed to the display. The individual must also have the ability to disassociate the movements of the eyes from the head. The person must be able to move the eyes from left to right, right to left without stopping in the midline, eyes up and eyes down, be able to affix the gaze on a specific target and shift that gaze. The individual will also need the motor control movement to either hit a switch or access directly with, for example, the hand or a pointer.
- *Motor planning.* The individual must be able to organise and carry out the specific task required.
- *Visual.* The individual must have sufficient visual acuity to see the display and the specific symbols/pictures on it.
- *Perceptual.* Visual discrimination of position and space, spatial relationships and figure ground are all important features in scanning.
- *Kinaesthetic.* To operate a switch effectively one must be able to hit the switch without looking at it so that the visual attention can be kept on the display.
- *Cognitive.* An individual must be able to remember where the required picture/icon is and must understand the task required to select it.

- *Linguistic.* The individual must be able to understand the instructions given so that the overall skill can be learnt and built upon.

Visual Tracking versus Visual Scanning

Cooke & Hussey (1995) describe visual tracking as the ability to follow a target with one's eyes, that is, where the object moves. Visual scanning is described as finding a specific visual target in a field of several targets, that is, that is the eyes move.

In order to decide on the most appropriate AAC system for an individual, visual tracking and visual scanning need to be assessed. Visual scanning normally develops at a young age, but individuals with physical disabilities may present with difficulties in any or all of the components involved.

Development of Visual Scanning

Young babies start developing visual scanning ability by watching people such as parents and siblings moving around in their environment, that is, tracking the person moving. As head control develops and improves, babies look at moving objects (visual tracking) and then use their visual scanning ability to look for objects which they want. A child will also look from one object to another, or at a specific object to make a choice.

Many children with severe disability are quite irritable when they are young babies. They are regularly carried by their parent for much of the day, often in a position which does not allow them to look around their environment for stimulation. Children with severe disability also have difficulty in lifting their head independently so that they do not gain the ocular motor control to follow objects or scan for what they want. These children are seldom given the opportunity to make choices either.

Children with physical disability require an increased number of opportunities to learn visual tracking and scanning. Some individuals may require a long time to learn the skill of visual tracking and scanning.

Summary

All the considerations discussed above cannot be treated separately when it comes to practical implementation. The areas need to be addressed in terms of the following general questions.

How do all these skills function together?
For example, an individual with relatively good language and symbolic skills may not be able to utilise these skills to his potential on an AAC system, if he cannot access that system. Therefore, while it is necessary to consider the skills separately (and this can help a lot in trying to determine which area is hindering progress), it is also necessary to analyse their functional use in combination. In this way, the abilities and needs of the individual are best met.

Is the individual motivated to use the system?
If an individual has relatively good skills in all areas but no desire to use the system, this means that these skills are not currently functional. In this case the clinician can gain an understanding of the individual's abilities which will highlight the reduced motivations as the issue. Motivation may have been deemed the main problem area prior to the AAC assessment. The process of assessment may serve, for example, to highlight a more specific problem eg, scanning, which has served to reduce the individual's motivation, or identify an individual for whom the expectations around AAC system use have been too high.

What is the individual's preference?
An individual may have relatively good skills but may not want a comprehensive or complex AAC system. For example, his goal for AAC may be for it to help him communicate only in certain situations. We know a significantly unintelligible adult who was fairly intelligible to her family and friends. Her desire was for a portable system that she could take to the pub to order drinks! This was provided and met her needs as determined by her.

What are the individual's other needs?
Does the AAC system need to meet other requirements such as environmental controls and word processing?

CHAPTER 4

The Functional Effects of Physical Disability

Introduction

There are many causes of physical disability and very many different diagnoses. When working with individuals with physical disabilities, it is important to have as much information as possible about the diagnosis. This allows the clinician to evaluate the current and future status of the individual and make recommendations concerning the prescription of equipment.

- Although many of the congenital physical disabilities are non-progressive, for example, cerebral palsy, the child's functional abilities will change as the child matures and interacts with the environment.
- The way in which the individual controls his body while interacting with the environment is of particular importance. The clinician must establish to what extent the physical disability is affecting the individual's development and functioning.
- The maturing child should be using all the senses – vision, hearing, kinaesthetic, vestibular, smell and taste – to explore his environment. The information returning through all the senses must be interpreted so that the child can respond to it. This produces an adapted response which can be modified and built upon. This is how the young child

develops the postural control to withstand gravity and interact in the environment. This process is interrupted by physical disability. The child may not be able to overcome gravity, or move his head without eliciting abnormal patterns of movement, or too much movement. Some children are very frightened by movement, especially quick movements. Their sensory feedback may be altered.

- Children with physical disabilities are often carried for much of the day. This may be for one or more of the following reasons:

  - The child has been in hospital for a long period.
  - The child is very irritable.
  - The child cannot tolerate a bed or a seat.
  - The parents are unable or are unwilling to let their child cry.

  If children with physical disability are carried continuously they may not have had the opportunity to develop postural control. They do not have the chance to interact with their environment. Learning opportunities are missed.

- Voluntary movement may be very difficult and unrewarding for the individual with a physical disability. For some, the more effort that is required, the more frustrated the individual becomes as muscle tone increases, or the opposite to the required movement is produced. For others, effort increases the involuntary movements and reduces postural stability. Some individuals require a longer time to process the incoming information and so there is a delayed motor response, or there may also be a delay in processing the response itself.

- Any of these difficulties make it difficult to pick up the signals the individual is trying to give. This may result in his efforts being ignored or misinterpreted. This is very discouraging for the individual and may result in them being unwilling to try again. Clinicians must be aware of this during evaluation, and not be too hasty in declaring that the individual is uncooperative, or perhaps even has a learning disability.

- Individuals with significant learning and physical problems may benefit from the multi-sensory assessment approach. The physical responses may be very subtle or very exaggerated and the clinician will need to observe closely.

- Individuals with a less severe disability may have poor sitting balance and may use their arms to prop themselves up. When given sitting support in a chair, the hand function may not be accurate enough to activate a target smaller than a large switch. Some individuals may have good gross upper limb control, but no independent finger control.

Postural Control

The background physical development for movement and stability is postural control. The clinician must be able to assess the:

- Postural control as the individual changes from the rest position to activity
- Effects of different positions on the postural control
- Effort involved in voluntary control and movement, and
- Speed at which the individual fatigues.

If an individual is not developing the postural control to sit and balance and hold his head up, the use of an AAC system will be affected.
    Postural control affects the following:

- The stability required to shift weight and move, eg, head, arm and leg.
- The stability required to sit, hold head up and move eyes, eg, look to a desired person.
- The stability required to control movements against gravity, eg, pressing a key on a keyboard without the arm/hand resting on the other keys, and then releasing the key.

Position

The position of the individual with a physical disability is important. The individual's postural control will differ depending on the position. On any given day an individual may be placed in/on some or all of the following positions: floor, side lying board, chair, stander, walker, buggy, car seat, bath, potty chair, person's arms. The amount of support required, and provided by the equipment will depend on the individual's postural control and the functional activity. For example, a child of six years with very low muscle tone centrally (trunk and neck) and high muscle tone distally (arms and legs), who uses spasticity to lift his head, may be best placed on the floor with his head and shoulders on a wedge for functional activities. This position should be utilised while a more age-appropriate position, for example, a custom-designed supportive seating system, is being made and trialled.

An individual's optimum position for function should produce the most controlled movement/s with the least amount of effort, to control the device. If a movement requires a lot of effort, the Bobath concept (see Figure 4.1) places the person with physical disability in a circle of diminishing returns.

Motor Control

The Characteristics of Movements
The characteristics of movements required for AAC are:

- Purposeful movement
- Repeatable movement
- Reliable movement
- Accurate movement
- Efficient movement

The movement may be of the eyes, for example, looking up to say 'yes', or of the head, arm, hand, knee, foot.

The individual may achieve a purposeful and repeatable movement but he may require training to establish the movement as a reliable, accurate and efficient one. It is important not to mount switches too quickly as the individual may experience failure or may be injured by the switch.

Changes in the Individual's Motor Control
As a child develops he changes. Furthermore, most children improve in motor control and refine their abilities with training. As a result of this, assessment for AAC is continuous, and equipment should be upgraded as abilities improve.

Children also grow and this may have a detrimental impact on the person's physical ability, for example, increased tightness (spasticity) with rapid growth spurts.

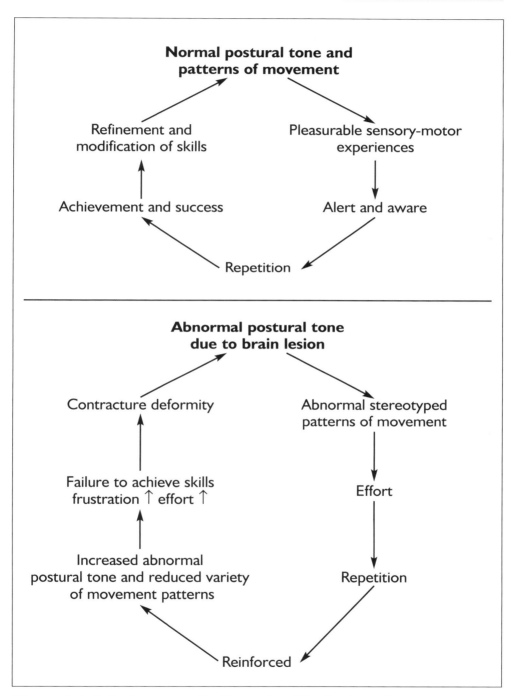

Figure 4.1 *Bobath concept: feedforward and feedback mechanisms*

The equipment the individual uses also needs to change and be adapted as the person develops. For example, a child may require greater support as he becomes taller and needs to change from a buggy to a wheelchair. A young child does not need the high level of accuracy required by the older child using more sophisticated systems.

- Initially the child may swipe at a switch to operate a toy with its hand.
- Greater postural control is necessary for accuracy on a scanning system, which places a high demand on the individual.
- A new movement is required.
- A new position for the switch may be necessary.

An individual with a deteriorating condition, such as leucodystrophy, will require re-evaluation as motor control deteriorates.

The Importance of Symmetry
When a movement has been found, it is important that the individual is positioned in a symmetrical position.

Many individuals have an asymmetrical distribution of tone, and one side, or one half of the body, is tighter than the other. If this is used functionally, the individual uses one side of the body in a tight, fixed position, so as to release the other side for use. One individual with athetosis whom we assessed looped one arm around the push handle of his wheelchair in order to give the trunk stability, and to free the opposite arm to operate an expanded keyboard.

In this asymmetrical position, the body is then placed as follows: one shoulder is forward, the head is turned to the side, the spinal column is rotated and this pulls the pelvis out of position and brings the hip forward on the same side as the shoulder. This reduces the base of support on the seat, which reduces the individual's stability. To compensate for this, the person must pull the legs into tight flexion to 'hang on' to the chair.

Over time, the individual may develop some or all of the following contractures – scoliosis of the spine, or subluxation or dislocation of the hip joint. The individual's sitting ability is reduced and he may also experience a great deal of pain. The individual may require surgery just to regain his sitting ability. A new method of accessing the device will also have to be found, as the initial movement was incorrect for this individual.

Use of Physical Disability as a Means to Communicate
Some individuals learn to use their high tone and spasms. They push into very strong extension as a way of saying no and avoiding working on directed activities. We often see children, and young teenagers, use this form of behaviour because of the frustration of not being able to communicate. This leads to great distress for the individual and the parents and carers.

Effective motor control does not follow on through use of increased muscle tone. It is important to work with these young children in supported positions in the therapist's, parent's and carer's arms. This facilitates the evaluation of the situations that trigger off this response, and how the individual initiates the extensor thrust.

With consistent good handling techniques and verbal cues the child can be facilitated to stop this behaviour while another more functional system of communication is established. While establishing postural support for functional symmetrical positions the child's head position is very important for ocular motor control and the use of vision.

Visual Difficulties
Some individuals with physical disabilities have problems with vision. There may be:

• Immaturity or damage to the optic nerves
• Loss of field of vision
• Acuity problems
• Blindness
• Squint, and
• Nystagmus.

It is important that the individual has an ophthalmic assessment, if concerns arise. The clinician, where possible, should discuss the findings of the assessment in relation to the individual's functional abilities. The ophthalmologist should be able to answer questions regarding the individual's vision.

The Mobility Issue

In AAC assessment there are significant differences when assessing an individual who is independently mobile, or mobile on crutches, and one who uses a wheelchair or walker.

- Individuals who walk or use crutches do not necessarily have good balance or good fine finger motor control.
- These individuals are unable to carry heavy devices and may not wish to give up their independent mobility for independent communication.
- The portability of devices has been an issue for a long time. Smaller and lighter devices are being designed but these require accurate functional access ability, or the use of an external switch. An external switch further reduces the portability.
- Portability is not so difficult for the individual who uses a wheelchair. The device can be mounted in the chair, as can a switch if required. When an individual uses a wheelchair for mobility the challenge may be to get the correct seating position and switch location. Care must be taken when mounting switches and devices that the individual and carers give their input to the final overall appearance. No one wants to look like a machine.

CHAPTER 5

Pre-Assessment

Introduction

The assessment sections in this manual are divided into different areas for use with particular individuals. Clinicians should use a combination of sections from different chapters *as appropriate to the individual's needs*. For example, the initial case history and information retrieval section is relevant to individuals who may go on to use either low- or high-tech communication systems. The section which relates to establishing 'Yes' and 'No' signals can relate to many types of individuals, whatever their needs.

Not all sections need to be used in the assessment process for the following reasons:

- The assessment process for AAC involves many areas and can be lengthy enough without adding unnecessarily to the duration or frequency of sessions.
- People with physical disabilities can tire easily due to the effort involved in physical or cognitive activities.
- We do not need to add to the frustrations of individuals unable to express themselves. We should be able to 'pick up' information during sessions without extended testing of all areas.
- The individual's needs should be relatively clear from the initial probes and information provided by carers and local service providers.

- Diagnostic therapy will often inform us more accurately than extensive and numerous assessments.

In other words, *assessments should be targeted to yield necessary and maximum information.*

The clinician should take into account factors relating to previous AAC systems, such as familiarity with a previous AAC system and symbols, success of the previous system, and the user's attitude to the previous system.

Considerations should be given to both high- and low-tech systems during the assessment process if the individual has the potential for a high-tech system. All individuals who may benefit from a high-tech communication aid should also have a low-tech system for the following reasons – it will be available as a back-up system should the communication aid break down and need to be repaired, and a low-tech system can function as a major resource for communication while the individual familiarises himself with the voice-output device.

Where an individual has both low- and high-tech systems, both should be compatible in terms of their organisation.

It is important to remember that the initial evaluation is not the be all and end all of the assessment process. This is particularly so in light of the following considerations:

- User needs may change for the better
- User needs may change for the worse
- Technology may become outdated, and
- The user's current system may have an irreparable fault.

It is important to remember to try to evaluate the *potential* of individuals as well as the *presence* of skills. With this in mind we find it best to include teaching as part of the assessment. The question asked is:

If an individual cannot do the task after a number of trials, can he learn to do it?

This is mainly because of the potentially limited linguistic experience of an individual who is physically disabled. This can happen despite intensive language therapy and the variety of activities a person is offered. Particularly important in language and communication development, we feel, is the ability to actually physically participate in the world and actively explore environments.

If there are dominating issues, for example, with regard to scanning or access then the clinician may want to administer activities in these sections first. In doing so, evaluations of the individual in other areas will be facilitated. This perspective of skills influencing each other and all needing to be accommodated will increase the reliability of the assessment process.

Tasks are criterion referenced and therefore measure the ability of the individual with reference to that particular task only. Examples of tasks are given to facilitate the clinician, but as they are criterion referenced, substitutions can be made by the clinician regarding content etc, with regard to the individual's motivations or skills.

The tasks/activities outlined are intended to sample communication skills rather than be a complete representation of a person's abilities. If the clinician is unhappy with the results obtained, perhaps because she is unsure of the consistency of the behaviour sampled, further tasks should be carried out to facilitate an understanding of the individual's skills. Not all activities in each section may need to be completed as the clinician may gain all the required information from a selected number of tasks.

Alternatives may be provided at the end of tasks to accommodate individual preference, give the clinician multiple choices for administering tasks, and to provide multiple tasks if reliability is an issue. Additionally, information from some of these tasks may have already been elicited by conducting tasks outlined in earlier chapters and these may not need to be carried out in light of this. The clinician should respond quickly to the individual's signals and responses to reinforce the behaviour.

Trial runs to demonstrate what is expected of the individual may be important with some individuals, particularly those with no or limited experience of AAC. Additionally, some individuals may need to be directly facilitated in the initial stages, for example, by placing their hand on the desired picture or object.

Pre-Assessment Forms

The aim of this pre-assessment stage is twofold:

1 To encourage the referral source and/or carer to evaluate clearly:

   - The individual's communication functioning
   - The reasons for referral, and
   - The individual's communication needs.

2 To provide the clinician with preliminary information on which to base accurate planning of the assessment.

Appointment Letter

This letter (Sample Form 1) provides the carers and local service providers with accurate and detailed information, and lays out the structure of the session.

Intake Form

This form (Sample Form 2) should be sent to the referral source and carers prior to the actual assessment, and should be seen as the initial step in the assessment process. The aim of the intake form is to retrieve:

- Identification information.
- Communication and AAC information.
- Reasons for referral. It is important to elicit a reason for referral as this can serve to highlight specific needs and motivations, for example, an individual moving to a new environment.
- Elicitation of the individual's likes and dislikes which can significantly aid in planning the assessment and in the accuracy of information obtained during that assessment.
- Information about the individual's functioning. Comprehension levels should ideally be established as much as is possible prior to the assessment process commencing.

Appointment Information
Speech & Language Therapy Department

Date

To

Address

Please note that an Augmentative and Alternative Communication Assessment has been arranged for:

Name

Address

DOB

further to a referral received from:

Name

Title

Address

This appointment has been organised for:

Day

Date

Time

and will last between 1 and 2 hours.

The assessment team present will be:

Speech & language therapist	Name
Other	Name
Other	Name
Other	Name

Please bring any relevant communication materials with you to the assessment. These may be communication boards and/or communication aids. Please confirm with us that you will be able to attend.

Secretary
Speech & Language Therapy Department
cc

Sample Form 1 *Appointment letter*

Intake Information
Identification details

Name _____

Address _____

_____

DOB _____

Medical diagnosis _____

_____

Hearing _____

Vision _____

Communication information

Comprehension
Most recent standardised results (if available)

_____

What are your informal observations?

_____

Expression
Most recent standardised results (if available)

_____

What are your informal observations?

_____

Speech
Comments

_____

Functional information

Hand Function

_____

Seating System

_____

Sample Form 2 *Intake form*

Other details

Please give results and dates of most recent:
Psychological testing

Reading and spelling abilities

Augmentative and Alternative Communication Information

1 Name this individual's primary carers at home and centre/school.

2 Name the professionals involved with this individual.

3 Note the primary communication environments.

4 Name the primary communication partners.

5 How does this individual currently communicate?

6 What are this individual's 'yes' and 'no' signals?

7 Has an augmentative and alternative communication (low- or high-tech) system been previously tried? If so, describe. Please include information on system type and programme/overlay.

8 How successful was this system? What contributed to its success or failure?

Sample Form 2 *continued*

9 Who has requested this assessment and for what reasons?

10 How does the individual feel about the referral? How do the primary carers feel?

11 What are the individual's requirements from this assessment?

12 What are the carer's requirements from this assessment?

13 What are the referral source's requirements?

14 Describe this individual's likes and dislikes.

15 Who will attend the assessment?

16 Please tick which reports you have enclosed.

☐ Speech & Language Therapy

☐ Occupational Therapy

☐ Medical

☐ Psychological

☐ Educational

☐ Physiotherapy

☐ Other ( )

Signed

Date

Sample Form 2 *Continued*

Communication Log

The Communication Log (Sample Form 3) will give the clinician information on important details such as:

- The individual's language/communication modes.
- The frequency of communications.
- The amount of initiations versus responses.
- The communication environments, and
- Communication needs.

It also serves another vital function. It encourages the person filling in the log (carer, parent) to focus on communication in general, and the communication of the individual in particular. This will mean the individual and others attending the session will come more prepared and more focused on the needs of the individual.

The AAC Needs Profile

This form (Sample Form 4) should be filled in by the speech & language therapist after discussion with the primary carer/s and the individual. It summarises information regarding AAC requirements and will help in planning and decision making. This type of approach actively encourages all those involved with the assessment process to determine what they want from it. It is open and relatively unstructured in order to reduce influence on those completing it.

Examples of possible answers are outlined below to facilitate an understanding of how this form can be used.

- *Features of system* – for example, portability, low cost, ease of programming, other facilities besides communication, literacy based, direct access, etc.
- *Settings required in (General)* – for example, pub, school, college, care home, take away, football match, bank, supermarket, hospital, hairdresser, disco, etc.
- *Settings required in (Specific)* – for example, restaurant: McDonalds, The Curry House, work canteen etc.

- *Speech functions* – for example, to request information, to gain attention, to greet, to order etc.
- *Speech functions specific to settings required* – for example,
  Restaurant: McDonalds 'A hamburger and small fries please'
  Hairdresser: The Wave 'Just a trim please'.

Communication Log

- Please fill in this log for

  Name ....

  Address ....

  ....

  ....

  DOB ....

- It is to be a record of how the above individual communicates. Try not to *interpret* communication behaviours; instead, write down *exactly* what you see.

- Please remember that many behaviours can be communications. Examples of this are vocalisations, eye signals, body signals, words, etc.

- The log should be filled in for at least five selected situations during the day, for example, Lunchtime, Reading, In the Kitchen, Playtime etc, so it may need to be completed by a number of people. Please find enclosed multiple copies to facilitate recording.

- Try to record on a 'typical' day that is, one involving situations that occur most days.

- Please return the communication log to the person listed below.

  ....

  ....

  ....

  ....

  ....

Thank you for your help.

Sample Form 3 *Communication log*

Communication Log

Name of individual _____

Date log recorded _____

Describe situation _____

Name of person completing form _____

Form number   1 / 2 / 3 / 4 / 5

Time	Communication Behaviour (What did s/he do?)	What preceded the communication? (Question/Nothing)	What did carer say/do in response to the communication?	Was the communication spontaneous or elicited?

Sample Form 3 *Continued*

AAC Needs Profile

Name of Individual
Date Completed
Completed by

Please write as much as you want in each section.

Do you require a low-tech (eg, communication board) or high-tech (eg, communication device) system or both?

Do you have anything specific in mind?

Area	Comments
System features	
For which settings generally is the system required?	
For which settings specifically (give names) is the system required?	
What kind of communications do you want the system for? For example: to tell a story, to order, to get attention, to greet people.	

Sample Form 4 *AAC needs profile*

Please give specific examples of what phrases or words the system needs to include.
Give as many examples as you want. Continue on the next page if necessary.

Place	Word/phrase

Signed

Date

Sample Form 4 *Continued*

CHAPTER 6

Carer Interaction

Introduction

Focusing on the Carer

The focus of the interactional analysis is on the carer. We often find that enhancing the carer's interaction with the individual will produce spontaneous improvements in the individual's communication, whether this be increased use of communication, development of intent, or development of refined communication.

This focus on the carer is important because communication does not occur in a vacuum and the person selected for this is usually the individual's main communication partner. Sometimes the carers can be so focused on the caring aspect of their interaction with the individual, that other considerations may be secondary due to very understandable issues such as time constraints and energy levels. Implementing changes, at times to entrenched behaviours, requires effort, even when simple recommendations are given such as:

Wait for a minute to give him time to respond

Interaction in Different Environments
In considering interactional style, particularly with respect to implementation, the clinician may want to consider evaluating a number of interactions in a number of environments. The environment is vital to successful prescription and implementation because it can make for optimal use of AAC. Environments can be classified as follows:

- *Main environments* For example, school, home, take-away, park, grandparents' house, etc.
- *Sub-environments – places* For example, sub-environments within the school including break-time, maths class, arrival at school, news time, swimming time, etc.
- *Sub-environments – people* For example, siblings, peers, relatives, therapists, care assistant, etc.

Interactional Analysis for Adults and Children
This session is not only applicable to children. Often adult users, who may or may not have had a history of AAC use, may have to deal with some of the same issues of interactional communication as children.

Interactional Problems
Some of the interactional problems which can become apparent from this type of analysis are:

- Reduced communication opportunities for the individual.
- Lack of understanding of the individual's communication signals.
- Reduced carer understanding of the carer-individual communication style.

Inhibitors and Contributors
The analysis of the interaction should focus on what is inhibiting or contributing to successful communication for the individual. This can be evaluated in terms of motivators within the communication interaction and low effort, that is, what facilitates the individual without demanding excessive physical effort.

Early Communication Skills

This session can also be used to evaluate the individual's early communication skills, such as intent or shared attention. If used in this way, it can also serve to reduce the need for direct probes to evaluate early skills. For example, observation of the interaction can confirm the presence of such skills as turn-taking, early language understanding and communicative intent.

Information Sharing

As with all parts of the assessment procedure, it is always advisable to share information with the carer (and individual). The information gained is not for the sole use of the clinician! In the case of interaction, this may need to be handled with special care, and always in the context of facilitating productive change, if necessary.

Preparation

Observation Room

The use of a video link or observation room will significantly facilitate the retrieval of information by the clinician. Leaving the carer and individual alone in a room can produce a much more accurate picture of the communication interactions and interactional style. Similarly, recording on a video will give the clinician time to evaluate the interaction at leisure.

Timing

A ten-minute session is usually more than sufficient to provide the clinician with an idea of the carer-individual interaction. Preferably, this should be videoed with only the carer and individual in the room, as discussed above.

Materials

The clinician should provide materials that will encourage natural and ease of interaction. For children these can include:

• A single-channelled voice output switch with a song or phrase on it
• Switch activated toys

- Books
- Building blocks
- Dolls
- Toy vehicles
- Bubbles, etc.

It is essential that not too many items are available; usually five items such as those mentioned above are acceptable. The items should be appropriate to the cognitive level and age of the individual. Older individuals will require more age-appropriate materials. Another alternative is for the carers to bring in a few familiar items themselves.

Rules
It is important to prepare the carer by explaining what you require from the session. However, it is also vital that the clinician does not go into too much detail, as it may encourage the carer or individual to 'perform' rather than act as in everyday situations. Advise the carer on the rationale and the specific details of the session.

1   Rationale
    That it is important for the clinician to understand how the communication partners communicate together in order to implement and assess for an AAC system.

2   Specifics
    - How long the session will last
    - That the clinician needs to get an idea of how both partners communicate, so the clinician will be watching the interaction and may take some notes
    - That materials have been provided and there are no restrictions on either how they use them or where they are in the room
    - That the carer is to act as naturally as possible in the circumstances – that is, as if they were playing or talking at home
    - That if they need to relax they can spend some time together in the room where they will be observed before the clinician starts observing

- That the clinician has no specific expectations of them ie, they are not expected to do anything in particular during the observation, and
- That they will be told when they can stop!

Analysing the Interaction

Use the Interaction checklist (Sample Form 5) to help in analysing the interaction between the carer and individual. The checklist is organised into four main parts:

1   *Carer responsivity*. How the carer responds to the individual's signals. Please note that with the individual who is physically involved, this can be more difficult for the carer given the reduced range available to the individual and the increased effort involved in communicating.
2   *Communication style of the carer*. This helps identify particular problem areas if present.
3   *Communication control*. How equally is the communication interaction shared?
4   *Interaction representation*. How does the session reflect the 'normal' interaction between the carer and individual? This last section should be completed with the carer by asking direct questions of the carer.

The clinician may want to transcribe the interaction to answer some specific questions such as 'Who did the most talking?' and for record-keeping purposes. This, however, is not essential and most questions can be answered through observation alone.

Interaction Checklist

Name ....

Date ....

A RESPONSIVITY

Questions	Comments
1 Did the carer position him/herself so that the individual could interact with him/her?	
2 Did the carer appear to understand the individual's physical signals? Were these acknowledged?	
3 Did the carer appear to understand the individual's facial signals? Were these acknowledged?	
4 Did the carer appear to understand the individual's vocal and verbal signals? Were these acknowledged?	

B STYLE

Questions	Comments
1 Was the carer's language appropriate to the receptive level and age of the individual?	
2 Was the carer intelligible in terms of articulation, voice and fluency levels?	
3 Was the carer's voice animated if this was appropriate, that is, did it succeed in grabbing the individual's attention?	
4 Was the speed of the carer's output appropriate?	
5 What was the carer's predominant utterance type (eg, questions, comments)?	

Sample Form 5 *Interaction checklist*

C CONTROL

Questions	Comments
1 Who did the most talking (communicating) – the carer or individual?	
2 Was the carer following the individual's lead?	
3 When the individual communicated successfully, was this followed through either by confirming the communication or acting upon it?	
4 Did the carer leave verbal space and time for the individual to respond and communicate?	
5 Who directed the session?	

D REPRESENTATION

These questions should be directed to the carer after the session is completed.

Questions	Comments
1 How did the session feel?	
2 Do you feel this session was representative of your everyday interactions?	
3 If not, how was it different?	
4 I'm now going to feedback on my observations. Please tell me if you agree or disagree with them and why.	

Signed

Sample Form 5 *Continued*

CHAPTER 7

Multi-Sensory Assessment

Introduction

The material in this section is based on the work of Coupe *et al* (1988) who were among the first to bring the importance of multi-sensory stimuli to the attention of professionals working with severely disabled individuals. They used the term Affective Communication Assessment. By definition, Affective Communication focuses on the reactions of individuals to the presentation of stimuli across a number of sensory modes and assesses their responses to it on an affective level. It is the very earliest level of evaluating responses and attempting to develop communication skills based on these responses. It is particularly useful for individuals with severe sensory or cognitive impairments. We have added a further sensory experience which can often elicit reactions – that is, movement (kinaesthesia).

Essentially, this technique attempts to elicit positive and negative reactions from the individual using stimuli from a number of sensory areas. The responses of individuals at severe impairment levels tend not by nature to be refined reactions or communications. Elicited behaviours can vary from extreme reactions to subtle ones. Examples of the more subtle behaviours include:

- Mouth opening
- Eyes widening

- Leg extending
- Smiling
- Brief eye contact

It is the responses which are important as they can tell us what materials and senses we can use with these clients to develop skills such as intention, shared attention and more refined communications. For example, an individual who demonstrates positive reaction to sound may be a candidate for a single-channelled voice-output switch. An individual who reacts strongly to tactile stimuli may respond to a programme focusing on utilising tactile stimuli. This information can be used as the starting point in an AAC system. For example, tactile objects can be used to develop a communication system. This can take many forms, for example, using a tactile board, placing tactile symbols on a communication aid (to help the individual recognise the function of the symbols with reference to communication), or using an E-Tran (Eye-Transfer/Eye Gaze) frame.

If intention and cause and effect skills are not yet developed, this information can help the clinician plan a programme focusing on receptive and associative skills. An example of this is using a stimulus as an antecedent to a favourite activity in a structured and consistent manner. By associating it with a favoured activity, the individual can then be facilitated to use it spontaneously – the commencement of an AAC system. Specific examples are:

- If an individual responds to sound, facilitated activation of that sound perhaps via a Bigmack® can be followed by a motivational activity such as hugging. Facilitation can be gradually removed as the individual learns to use and associate the stimuli correctly.
- For an individual who enjoys movement, such as a motion activity like rolling, this can be used as a reward after touching an object only associated with that activity – that is, used as an antecedent to the activity. In this way the child can learn to use symbols to request activities.

Multi-sensory analysis has major bonuses:

- We develop an understanding of what can be motivating and aversive for an individual.
- We develop an understanding of what stimuli will elicit a response from him, enabling us to extend his repertoire of behaviours.
- We can plan specific programmes in a number of ways including:
  - Presenting stimuli which produce negative reactions to facilitate a more refined negative communication behaviour.
  - Using favoured activities to produce and develop refined positive communications.
  - Using specific stimuli to teach association (receptive skills) as a way to structure the routine for the individual, or as a precursor to work on expressive skills.

To be effective this type of programme needs to be highly structured. The individual, in other words, needs clear boundaries, antecedents and consequences in order to learn that it is the stimulus which produces the object or activity of his desire.

This type of analysis is often used as a basis for introducing tactile objects and objects of reference to an individual. Although the definitions of both can be similar, we prefer to define them separately as follows:

- *Tactile objects* are stimuli which are definable by touch but do not necessarily relate concretely to the object/activity they are being associated with for communication purposes.
- *Objects of reference* can be accessed tactilely or by eye referencing and bear a relationship to the item they are being used to communicate about. For example, a washcloth for bathtime or a cup for drinking. In using this type of analysis and when implementing communication systems based on the information retrieved, the clinician may need to be aware of those individuals who are tactile defensive.

Preparation

The clinician should prepare a range of stimuli for each sensory area as it can be difficult to predict in advance an individual's reaction. These stimuli should be designed to elicit negative, positive and neutral reactions. Therefore, ideally there should be two stimuli per sense (eg, touch) and per expected reaction (eg, negative). Therefore, for each sense, six stimuli at least should be available for presentation, although they may not all be used.

As some individuals at this level present with delayed responding behaviour and reduced reactions, stimuli should be potent, and presented:

- *A number of times.* When a stimulus is presented it can be withdrawn and re-presented to check for consistency of behaviour and accuracy of interpretation.
- *For longer periods than normal.* For example, if a stimulus does not elicit an immediate reaction, it should not be removed but held in place for a while. Up to one to two minutes is advisable in some cases for the individual to habituate.

Table 7.1 is a checklist to help in recording observations. However, the Multi-sensory stimuli assessment form itself (Sample Form 6) has blank spaces for the clinician to fill in. This is because the range of stimuli available to individual clinicians can vary, as can the stimuli which are motivating to particular individuals. Clinicians should try to use familiar stimuli in addition to unfamiliar ones. The information which will make planning easier can be elicited in advance of the actual assessment. Examples of this may be tunes from a favourite video, sounds which elicit activities he enjoys such as water running for a bath.

Before presenting stimuli, it is important to ensure it is safe to do so and confirm that there will be no allergic or harmful reactions. Prior to letting a child taste food, the clinician should check it is all right to do this. Following safety and hygiene procedures is crucial. For example, always using a glove and spatula for presenting items. And remember, a tiny amount is usually enough to elicit a reaction.

The clinician should ensure a non-distracting environment is used so that responses can be paired with the stimuli presented and reliably and accurately interpreted. Multiple stimuli should not be provided simultaneously. Each stimulus should be selected for its uniqueness as

Table 7.1 *Examples of multi-sensory stimuli*

Auditory stimuli

Positive	Neutral	Negative
Music of favourite video/ television programme	Classical music	Clapping
Tape of carer's voice	Clock	Heavy metal music
Rattle	Water running	Loud shouting
Drum	Kettle boiling	Stamping feet
Car starting		Dog barking
Telephone ringing		Vacuum cleaner

Visual stimuli

Positive	Neutral	Negative
Picture of favourite character	Sheet of neutral coloured paper	Pen torch
Sheet of red paper	Adult book with neutral cover	Black-and-white striped paper
Photograph of mother	Balloon	Spiky ball
Favourite video (without sound)	Plant	Lighted candle
Christmas lights	Work surface material	Mirror
Bubbles		

Olfactory stimuli

Positive	Neutral	Negative
Chocolate drink	Plant leaf	Nail polish
Home-made dinner	Soil	Vinegar
Orange juice	Coffee	Perfume
Crisp	Tea	Bleach
	Baby food	

Tactile stimuli

Positive	Neutral	Negative
Touch to hand	Block of wood	Bubble wrap
Cotton	Vinyl	Rice
Silk	Placemat	Ice
Felt	Table surface	Sandpaper
Water	Sand	Corduroy material
Playdough	Bean bag	Screw
Sand	Regular surfaced toy	Spiky ball
		Sticky tape

continued

Table 7.1 *Continued*

Gustatory stimuli

Positive	Neutral	Negative
Chocolate spread	Baby food	Mustard
Crisp	Porridge	Vinegar
Favourite treat	Natural yoghurt	Coffee
Sugar	Cheese	Lemon juice
Honey	Ice-cream	Grapefruit

Kinaesthetic stimuli

Positive	Neutral	Negative
Rolling	Holding	Jumping
Slow swinging	Walking with individual	Quick movements
Hugging	in arms	

much as possible. For example, if the clinician is presenting a neutral taste such as baby food or porridge, it should not be lumpy to rule out a reaction to texture and maintain the sanctity of the response and the clinician's ability to interpret it. The clinician should be careful when performing the kinaesthetic tasks with individuals with physical disability as they can elicit abnormal postural tone.

Stimuli Examples

To decide what specific stimuli to utilise, the clinician should learn about the individual's likes and dislikes and look around her own environments. There are many things in the environment which can be used without modification. It is important to note that reactions to stimuli vary from individual to individual. What will be neutral for one person may be negative for another.

Multi-Sensory Stimuli Assessment

Name _____ **Date** _____

Write down the name of the exact stimulus before you present it. Chart the individual's specific response to the presentation of each stimulus. Then analyse whether the response can be interpreted as positive, neutral or negative.

Stimulus	Describe response	Positive	Neutral	Negative	No response
Auditory Positive 1 2 Neutral 1 2 Negative 1 2					
Visual Positive 1 2 Neutral 1 2 Negative 1 2					
Tactile Positive 1 2 Neutral 1 2 Negative 1 2					
Olfactory Positive 1 2 Neutral 1 2 Negative 1 2					

Sample Form 6 *Multi-sensory stimuli assessment*

Stimulus	Response	Positive	Neutral	Negative	No response
Gustatory Positive 1 2 Neutral 1 2 Negative 1 2					
Kinaesthetic Positive 1 2 Neutral 1 2 Negative 1 2					

Summary 1 – Responding Behaviour

Describe positive responding behaviour

Describe neutral responding behaviour

Describe negative responding behaviour

Sample Form 6 *Continued*

Summary 2 – Senses

	Sense	Stimulus
Positive		
Neutral		
Negative		

Signed _____

Sample Form 6 *Continued*

CHAPTER 8

Establishing Basic Skills

Introduction

Very often the primary carers are so accustomed to the individual and his needs that they habitually understand what he wants, or his likes and dislikes. Their experience of the individual is important, but in cases like this it follows that the communication opportunities for the individual can be limited. This is due to anticipatory behaviour on the part of the carers which reduces the need to communicate even on a needs level. This of course limits the development of intentional communication, shared attention and refined communication behaviours.

This is by no means an attempt to comprehensively evaluate early communication skills which, as already discussed, are essential to the successful implementation of AAC systems. Instead it is intended to provide an overview of the individual's functioning to help in determining the basic skills an individual brings to the assessment process, and to facilitate the clinician in organising this.

Assessment Areas

Basic Communication Skills

Guidelines

The speech & language therapist is well informed about informal procedures for assessing basic communication skills. These can be readily assessed through an informal chat with the individual, primary carer and other service providers, and through observation of the individual. Alternatively, the clinician may want to use specific probes. For example, for shared attention and communication intent, blowing bubbles is usually a winner. Does the individual look at the bubble to request more? Does he attend to the activity? Does he make eye contact with the clinician? Examples of basic skills are:

- Shared attention
- Intentional communication
- Physical posture and tone.

Physical posture is included in this section because of the close relationship between physical and communication skills in the physically disabled population. The clinician needs to evaluate communication and other developmental areas in the context of the impact of physical development on these areas.

The clinician can assess other skills which she feels are essential for an understanding of the individual using the Basic communication skills observation sheet (Sample Form 7). For a comprehensive overview of an individual's skills, the therapist should utilise measures such as the Pre-Verbal Communication Schedule (Kiernan & Reid, 1997), Receptive Expressive Emergent Language Test (REEL) (Bzoch & League, 1991), The Pragmatics Profile of Everyday Communication Skills in Children (Dewart & Summers, 1995), or the Communication and Symbolic Behaviour Scales (Wetherby & Prizant, 1993).

This section can be absorbed easily into the introductory part of the session, and an idea of these behaviours can be elicited by questions to the individual and confirmatory questions to the carer and professionals. Alternatively, it can be incorporated into the interaction session, which, if videoed, can be evaluated at leisure by the clinician.

Multiple probes and carer's observations can confirm the consistency and reliability of behaviours observed during the session. It is important to establish these parameters and this can be achieved with:

- *Open questions* such as: 'How does he communicate for something he wants?'
- *Confirmatory questions* such as: 'He does like ice-cream doesn't he?'

Basic Communication Skills Observation Sheet

Name _____ **Date** _____

Skill	Behaviour	Physical Observations	Carers' Comments
Physical posture and tone			
Shared attention			
Communicative intention			
Other			

Signed _____

Sample Form 7 *Basic communication skills observation sheet*

Task examples

Skills can be probed in an informal manner either by observation or direct probes.

Shared attention/orientation to communication. Information on this aspect of communication can be elicited, for example, by:

- Directed commands such as:

  > 'Look at Mummy' or 'Show me your leg'.

- Utilising an activity which is highly motivating to the individual, for example, blowing bubbles.
- Referencing a person or item in the room and commenting on it, for example:

  > 'Look, there's a dog!' or 'You have a blue shoe. I have a red shoe.'

- Talking about a favourite character or activity of the individual, for example, a television character.
- Using an age-appropriate book and commenting on the pictures.
- Using the individual's photographs or photo pictures, such as ColorCards™, and commenting on them.

Intent. Intent will usually be observed as a result of the above activities.

- Favourite and despised foods can usually elicit a reaction and yield intentional behaviours. For example:

  > 'I love to eat snails. I hear you do too!
  > No? Do you like ice-cream?'

Photographs or comments can be used depending on the individual.

- A desirable object such as a battery-operated toy animal can be demonstrated and then partially hidden. Wait for the individual to request it.
- Similarly, the carer can be asked to leave the room. Comment on the leaving and wait for the individual to request, in whatever way he can, the return of that person.

- Place a toy or item in sight of the individual but out of reach. Wait for him to request it. Commenting on it may facilitate his attention and encourage a response.

Physical posture and tone. To evaluate for physical posture and tone, the clinician should note the starting position and any changes observed. This can be done while the individual is involved in activities.

Basic Communication Skills Examples

The checklist in Table 8.1 gives the clinician an idea of what type of entries can be made on the Basic communication skills observation sheet

Table 8.1 *Basic communication skills checklist*

Skill	Behaviour	Physical Observations	Carers' Comments
Physical posture and tone	Position at rest Postural changes Tonal changes Involuntary movements	Head is down Extensor thrust when lifting head	Mother reports this is typical
Shared attention	Listens to talking Makes eye contact to person when talking Smiles at reference to self Makes appropriate facial expressions	Stills Looks at person talking but this is brief due to inability to hold head up When named, smiles	Mother reports he can share attention by laughing, using his eyes to look at people
Intentional communication	Looks at object Greets Responds to commands by trying to touch Uses gestures	Unable to hold gaze successfully due to instability Turns to person entering Reaches for object with increased tone Tone increases	Speech & language therapist reports he looks at objects or pictures of things he wants or to convey information
Other			

(Sample Form 7). It should be used to formally record the behaviours observed, the carer's observations etc. This will help to identify the presence of these skills.

Communication Modes Form

This form (Sample Form 8) which should be filled in by the speech & language therapist, can be used to help in evaluating the modes the individual uses to communicate. It will give some idea of the preferred mode of the individual, or if AAC systems are already in place, the actual use of the system. Ideally, the session should be videoed and analysed at a later time. In this way the clinician can be sure of not missing any signals the individual may be using.

As the information obtained can be affected by the person the individual is communicating with and the type of interaction, the clinician is best to approach retrieval of information in this section in two main ways:

- Observation of individual–carer interaction as outlined in Chapter 6. The video of this session can be used to analyse basic communication skills too. Alternatively, the clinician can observe the individual in a familiar setting. In this case, the observation should last between 30 and 60 minutes, if the most reliable and maximum amount of information is to be retrieved.
- As the individual will be communicating with a familiar partner in the above scenario, it may be advantageous to observe interaction with an unfamiliar partner to probe the breadth of communication modes used, and to administer small tasks if the objective of the session has not been achieved. Tasks which will facilitate retrieval of information on the use of communication modes include those typically utilised by speech & language therapists. For example, daily activities, picture naming, picture description and conversation. The observations should be noted on the Communication modes form (see Sample Form 8).

Early Developmental Skill Probes

In some cases, the clinician may need to directly probe for the early developmental skills which have been discussed in previous chapters. For example:

Communication Modes Form

Name _____ **Date** _____

Mode	Number of times used	Proportion of total use (%)	Comments re success of mode/act
NO TECH Facial expression Head movements Proximal Gestures Signs Other			
LOW-TECH Pictures Symbols Other			
HIGH-TECH Single-channel switch Communication aid Other			
NATURAL VOICE Vocal Consonant + Vocal Single word Multi-word Other			

FAMILIAR AND UNFAMILIAR COMMUNICATION PARTNERS

Which communication modes are used predominantly with a *familiar* communication partner?

Which communication modes are used predominantly with a *unfamiliar* communication partner?

Signed _____

Sample Form 8 *Communication modes form*

- *Cause and Effect.* To probe this skill, the clinician could, for example:
  - Use a battery operated toy attached to a switch
  - Use a Bigmack® voice-output switch with a song or message from the carer recorded on it
  - Use skittles and a ball
  - Use bubbles

- *Problem solving.* To probe this skill, the clinician could use some of the following:
  - Shape sorters
  - Jigsaw puzzles, preferably large pieces with handles if the individual is physically disabled
  - Overtly hiding interesting toys behind pieces of cardboard. This can be done directly in front of the individual if they are physically disabled, or in a far corner of the room
  - Use two to three Bigmack® voice output switches. The clinician can place a favourite message (eg, 'I love . . . football team') or song on only one and demonstrate. She should place the array in front of the individual and wait while he tries to find the switch that activates the message.

Some of the early developmental skills, for example, turn-taking, decision making and task sequencing are covered in other areas, particularly in Chapter 13. Many of these skills can be described as both developmental and communicative in nature. Some individuals will need demonstration of activities first before understanding how they work. Other individuals may need facilitation of the motor response, for example, by placing their hand on a switch to activate a toy. Performance in all skills areas should always be interpreted with relevance to the individual's chronological and cognitive ages.

CHAPTER 9

Confirmation and Negation Signals

Introduction

Establishing 'Yes' and 'No' signals should be concurrent with advising communication partners not to rely solely on this kind of interaction with the individual. Too often we have seen AAC individuals reach adulthood with carers communicating only by asking questions which elicit a 'Yes' or 'No' signal from the person. A system of communication which relies on these signals only:

- Is not shared communication
- Is in the control not of the individual but of the communication partner
- Can significantly hinder the development of a more refined way of communicating
- Can limit the information the individual can convey.

We usually find that most individuals who attend for AAC assessment have 'Yes' and 'No' signals established to a degree. They may not be refined and consistent behaviours, such as saying 'No' or eyes up for 'Yes'. However, the carer usually is able to identify the signals. An example of less refined signals may be:

- Crying with a certain tone to indicate 'No'

- Vocalisation to indicate 'Yes', or
- Physical withdrawal for 'No'.

There are many occasions when individuals attending for assessment are reported to have the confirmation and negation signals developed. On assessment, however, the clinician may find that several different responses are being interpreted as 'Yes' and 'No'. Therefore, it is possible to see individuals who are reported to have these signals developed but who in fact do not use reliable (that is, consistent and repeatable) signals.

Many individuals with physical disability need time to organise the physical response. This needs to be considered in the context of assessing and recommending movement for signals. Establishing and implementing 'Yes' and 'No' signals is not the be all and end all of intervention. It may take a secondary role to more important considerations, for example, the development of eye-pointing skills. The absence of refined 'Yes' and 'No' signals does not preclude the potential for developing these skills through training.

Establishing Confirmation and Negation Signals

Guidelines
The clinician should be happy with the demonstrated signals when:

- Reliability for interpretation is fine
- The consistency of the signal is good, and
- The effort involved for the individual is not considerable in terms of time needed to produce the signal, energy required, and its impact on positioning and stability. When this is the case, there is no need to go through the whole checklist (Sample Form 9). In a number of cases, two simple directions are sufficient. These are:

'Show me your "Yes" '

and

'Show me how you say "No" '

Confirmation and Negation Signals Checklist

Name _____ **Date** _____

Carer Questions
1   Does the individual have a 'Yes' signal?
2   Describe it please.
3   Does the individual have a 'No' signal?
4   Describe it please.

Thank you for that information. Now please bear with me while I ask a couple of questions myself.

Question	Response	Postural and Tonal Changes
1 Can you show me how you say 'Yes'.		
2 Can you show me how you say 'No'.		

'That was great. Let's move on to something else now' (signals reliable).
or
'That was great. I am going to ask a few more questions now' (signals unreliable).

Question	True Response	Actual Response	Postural and Tonal Changes
Is your name *(false name)*?	N		
Is your name *(true name)*?	Y		
Am I your mother?	N		
Is this person *(true)* your mother?	Y		

Sample Form 9 *Confirmation and negation signals checklist*

Question	True Response	Actual Response	Postural and Tonal Changes
Is this a cup? (Show picture of a cup)	Y		
Is this a spoon? (Show picture of a ball)	N		
Is this a book? (Show book)	Y		
Is this a book? (Show doll)	N		
Are you a boy?	Y/N		
Are you a girl?	Y/N		
Tell me 'Yes' when I say the word 'banana' … book, school, banana.	Y		
Tell me if I say the word 'wheelchair' blue, car, kitchen.	N		
Do you like music?	Y/N		
Do you like television?	Y/N		

Summary
Is the 'Yes' signal reliable/interpretable?   Is the 'Yes' signal consistent/repeatable?   Is the 'Yes' signal efficient (not requiring too much effort)?   Identify the 'Yes' signal or potential signal.
Is the 'No' signal reliable/interpretable?   Is the 'No' signal consistent/repeatable?   Is the 'No' signal efficient (not requiring too much effort)?   Identify the 'No' signal or potential signal.

Signed _____

Sample Form 9 *Continued*

Confirmation and Negation Signals Checklist
If the individual is not able to demonstrate his confirmation and negation signals in response to the above, the Confirmation and negation signals checklist (Sample Form 9) on the previous pages should be used. This will facilitate evaluation of the consistency, reliability and viability of these signals.

'Yes' and 'No' Trials: Non-Verbal and Early Verbal Signals

Guidelines
With some individuals it will be obvious that 'Yes' and 'No' signals are not established because the individual has not reached that level of functioning. If this is the case, the clinician should consider Multi-Sensory Analysis.

There are times when the clinician will need to discard, develop or help create new 'Yes' and 'No' signals. This can be for reliability, consistency or efficiency purposes or because of physical restrictions. The clinician should be wary of utilising any abnormal patterns such as flexion with spasticity of the upper arm. There are implications for increased tone and contractions in utilising such patterns. If this is the case, a number of trials should be carried out focusing on the most likely modes to convey these signals. These are outlined in Sample Form 10.

Depending on the level of functioning of the individual, the clinician may need to demonstrate the actions required. Due to the nature of physical disability, the clinician who is conducting this section may need to give the individual multiple opportunities to practise. This will help the clinician establish the potential for use of the signals.

Non-Verbal and Early Verbal Signals Checklist
The 'Yes' and 'No' trials have been broken down into two sections, non-verbal and early verbal signals, and facilitated signals.

The clinician should check non-verbal signals first because they are more independent, and potentially more reliable signals. If this is not successful, then the section focusing on facilitated signals should be attempted.

Confirmation and Negation Signals
Non-Verbal and Early Verbal Trials Checklist

That was good. Now I am going to see if we can try and make another 'Yes' and 'No'.

Trial	Describe Response
Head Nod Shake Turn right Turn left	
Arm/Hand Raise your right (*this side*) arm Raise your left arm Raise your right hand Raise your left hand Can you move any fingers? Raise this finger Raise this finger	
Facial Smile (*like this*) Frown Raise your eyebrows Lower your eyebrows Open your mouth Close your mouth	
Eye Look up Look down Look to the right Look to the left	
Leg/Foot Lift your right leg Lift your left leg Lift your left foot	

Sample Form 10 *Confirmation and negation signals: non-verbal and early verbal trials checklist*

Trial	Describe Response
Leg/Foot	
Lift your right leg	
Lift your left leg	
Lift your left foot	
Lift your right foot	
Move your right leg outwards (*towards me*)	
Move your right leg inwards (*towards your other leg*)	
Move your left leg outwards	
Move your right leg inwards	
Move your right foot outwards	
Move your right foot inwards	
Move your left foot outwards	
Move your left foot inwards	
Voice	
Say 'Yes'	
Say 'No'	
Say 'ah'	
Say 'oh'	
Say …	

Summary
What are the potentially useful 'Yes' signals?
What are the potentially useful 'No' signals?
Are there any movements produced which are contraindicated ie, using abnormal patterns?

Signed

Sample Form 10 *Continued*

'Yes' and 'No' Trials: Facilitated Signals

Guidelines
If the clinician is not able to establish reliable confirmation and negation signals, it may at this point be worth trialling basic switches and symbols which may provide the motivation to overcome the effort required for those individuals for whom it is physically difficult.

Switches
The clinician should first look at whether the individual:

- Can access the switch
- How he accesses it (see Chapter 14), and
- If it is motivational for him.

Then she should decide where to place the switches, for example, on a tray, near the head, on the left or right sides, etc. A number of locations may need to be trialled. The clinician should use a single channelled voice output switch such as the Bigmack®. If the individual cannot directly access this, the clinician may need to attach it to a smaller switch to facilitate access such as the Jelly Bean®, Specs® or Lolly® switch. A message should be recorded on to the switch. This message can be as simple as:

> 'Hello'
> or
> 'My name is ...'

If possible, the message should be recorded using a familiar voice, preferably that of the carer. Songs or music can also be recorded on to the switch depending on what is motivating to the individual. The idea here is just to see whether the individual has the concept of cause and effect (important for switch and communication use), and whether he will respond to voice output.

The next stage is to see if the individual can use a switch for a confirmatory or negatory purpose. The clinician should record either signal on to the switch and use a question such as:

'Is your name … ?'

If the individual is able to select pictures, the clinician should use pictures to elicit these responses. For example:

'Is this a cup?'

The clinician may want to demonstrate this first, and may also need to facilitate the individual in activating and utilising this to help him understand the process.

The clinician can then see if the individual can use two switches and, if so, can he use them reliably for 'Yes' and 'No' responses? The next step is to evaluate whether it is possible to find a second switch point and then to trial the two switches. The first switch should preferably be green (for 'Yes'), with the second switch being red (for 'No').

If use of switches is deemed the most suitable system for 'Yes' and 'No' signals, a number of points should be considered:

- Out of preference for neatness and because trays are typically used for a number of functions, we tend to attach the Bigmack® voice-output switches to either sides of the wheelchair with the access switches placed on the tray or head supports (depending on switch points).
- We typically place the appropriate 'Yes' and 'No' symbols – either face pictures or colour-coded squares on to the access switch (eg, Jelly Bean®) or main switch (eg, Bigmack®). This helps with the communication partner's understanding of the use of the switches, and also with association training, so the individual can learn to associate more concrete symbols with communication (and hopefully use it in line with learning a more refined system).

Symbols

As with the switches, the location points and access points should be predetermined by a number of trials. This can be done via ordinary materials such as pieces of coloured cardboard. If the individual is using touch (direct access), the symbols may be placed on a tray in front of him appropriate to his range of movement, etc. If the individual is using eye pointing, then an E-Tran frame can also be used. This is made of perspex and can be purchased or made, for example, by seating departments/technicians. While any dimension can be used, a typical size is a frame of two feet square. A square hole is cut in the middle so that the individual and partner can see each other through it, from opposite sides of the frame. Symbols are attached to the frame with velcro. Duplicates are attached to the partner's side so the partner can follow the individual's eye pointing accurately. If the symbols can be recognised, then integration of these on to a communication board/folder should be considered. If the individual is able to recognise pictures, colour coding may not be needed. Similarly, if the individual can recognise writing, the pictures are inappropriate.

By this stage, the clinician will have gained some idea of the ability of the individual and will not need to proceed through all stages and levels. The checklist for the facilitated trials of confirmation and negation signal appears in Sample Form 11.

Confirmation and Negation Signals
Facilitated Trials Checklist

Name _____ **Date** _____

Switches

1 ACCESS

- Can the person access the switch directly?
- If so, which part of the body is most reliable and consistent (the switch point)?
- If the switch cannot be accessed directly, does a smaller switch help?
- If so, which part of the body is most reliable and consistent (the switch point)?
- Can two switches be used simultaneously?

2 LOCATION

- State exactly where each switch should be placed.
- Can the switches be velcroed onto the chair?
- If not, do they need to be mounted?
- Where, and how?
- If switches are deemed appropriate, who will be responsible for installing them?

3 MESSAGE

- Is the person hitting the switch reliably to elicit the message contained on the switch?
- Is use of the switch random or is there intent involved? (For example, does he wait until the message is finished before starting again?)
- Can the individual use the switches reliably to respond to 'Yes' and 'No' questions?
- Can the individual make choices using the switches (for example, between onions and chocolate?)

4 TRAINING

- Does the individual respond to direct facilitation of use of the switch?
- Would a period of training be necessary?
- Specify the area this training would focus on (for example, access, association etc.)
- Are switches recommended for this individual?
- If, so specify the details.

Sample Form 11 *Confirmation and negation signals: facilitated trials checklist*

Symbols

1 ACCESS
- Can this person access the symbols directly or should they be accessed via eye pointing?
- Where should the symbols be placed for easiest access?
- Can the individual scan from one symbol to another?

2 LEVELS OF REPRESENTATION
- Which symbolic level is the individual able to understand?
- Can the individual use these symbols communicatively that is, can he answer 'Yes' and 'No' questions using them?

3 SIZE
- What size symbol can the individual reliably use?

4 TRAINING
- Is the individual able to use the symbols immediately or is further training required?
- Will these symbols stand alone or can they be integrated into a system such as an E-Tran frame or a communication board?

Signed _____

Sample Form 11 *Continued*

Chapter 10

Positioning

Assessment of Seating Position

The goal when positioning an individual with physical disabilities for communication systems is to provide the most functional position for the individual which is comfortable and safe.

The upright position facing forwards, and in midline is the optimum position for communication, but it is not exclusive. People communicate in all positions and environments, for example, on the floor, standing, in the bath, in the classroom. There are a wide variety of commercial devices available for persons with a physical disability to facilitate function, comfort and safety, for example, side lyers, buggies, car seats, walkers, wheelchairs. Individuals with physical disabilities will need assessment for the most appropriate equipment, and often the pieces of equipment require customisation. It is important to remember that no one piece of equipment will suit all situations. As the person changes and the environments he frequents change, the equipment must be re-evaluated.

It can be difficult to get the positioning correct for individuals with severe physical disability. As the upright position is considered important for breathing, communication, feeding and digestion, it is usually the first to be assessed. It will take more than one session to be achieved, and even with many fittings and trials, any change, for example, in the person's health, growth, or point of access to a communication device, can render the positioning of equipment inappropriate.

There are a number of basic principles which can be applied, but it will take practice and experience to come up with some of the creative solutions which may be required. The whole team's input is necessary to produce an effective result.

Assessment of Position

The following questions need to be addressed when considering what is an optimal position for an individual.

- How does the individual function without any intervention?

  - Can he look at toys, touch a toy, grasp/release?
  - Can he move, sit, change position?
  - How are the above achieved: with/without assistance, with/without abnormal movements/tone?

- Does the individual require preparation for functional movements? Does the environment require preparation?

  - What is the reaction to loud sounds, sudden movements, slow movement?
  - Has he very tight muscle tone in his body, limbs? Can this be changed and how?
  - Is there a difference in the reaction to hard and soft surfaces?

- Where is the position of least amount of support provided by the therapist's hands, which gives the most stability and functional ability?

  - Can the person achieve an upright position with the therapist's support?
  - Where is the therapist providing the support and how much?
  - Where does the individual have no tolerance to support?
  - Is more support needed to allow use of hands, head movements? Can these be achieved?
  - Can the optimal position be found where involuntary movements can be controlled or diminished?

- The clinician should try a functional activity in this position and assess its real usefulness, for example, operating a toy or food-mixer with a switch.
  - Can the position be maintained, or does tone become increased or fatigue set in with time?
  - Does the position allow movement, while maintaining or returning to original position?
  - Is the individual comfortable?
  - Is the individual safe? Will the position maintain range of movement or could contractures occur?
  - Is this position suitable, but for short periods only? Can the time be increased upon?

If the individual experiences difficulties with the position when being held by the clinician, either through increase in tone or involuntary movements, he can have great problems accommodating to the less pliable seating materials which cannot be sensitive to his fluctuating muscle tone.

Assessment of Seating System

The best positions found by the clinician and accurate body measurements should be noted. She should ensure seat depth, width and back height, are correctly set. The seat should be set to back (pelvic tilt) angle especially if this is difficult to change, and the footrests should be correct for knee and ankle measurements. It is important to give support to the pelvis first, the base should be firm but not hard. The clinician should then consider the following:

- Can the person be positioned comfortably sitting fully back into the seat with upper legs relaxed (not internally or externally rotated)? Is the pelvis level?
- A pelvic strap must be fitted which can be operated with one hand so that the other hand maintains position. This should be fitted at a 45° angle from the seat to ensure it is providing pelvic and hip stability.
- Is it necessary to place a block (pommel) in between the legs/knees to stop them internally rotating? This is not intended to hold the person into the seat.

- Is the pelvis stable or are further blocks/supports required at the sides to provide symmetry?
- Is a more contoured/closer fitting seat required for greater ability? A compromise may be necessary for people with involuntary movements as they cannot cope with prolonged confinement.
- Is the seat depth correct? When using contoured or ramped seats, there must still be space for knee flexion.
- What angle should the footrest be at? If an angle of greater than 90° is used, the individual with tight hamstrings will have great difficulty maintaining a neutral pelvic tilt. Most people require footrests at 90° to allow the feet to act as support in sitting.
- Can the individual place his feet flat on the footrests and take weight through them?
- Will angled footrests and/or foot straps assist with weight bearing?
- Can the person tolerate foot straps or heel cups with toe straps?

While observing the individual's position as the pelvis is being made stable, secure and symmetrical, the clinician must also observe the upper body. Again, the notes taken on how the individual managed when being held by the clinician will give starting pointers for the chair supports. The following questions should be considered:

- When the clinician supports the individual, what position of the trunk gives the best head control?
- Can the individual tolerate a straight, firm back support?
- Does the individual have any spinal abnormalities which require accommodation?
- Does a lumber pad help maintain the pelvic tilt and an erect spine?
- Will lateral supports on either side of the trunk provide the same support as the clinician's hands? How high up do they need to be?
- Was the individual able to use hands for function or are the upper limbs necessary for support, especially for head control?
- Is a head support device required? How much head support? Can it be provided without occluding range of vision?
- Does tilting the whole seating system improve or worsen the situation?

- Does the use of anterior support – chest strap, bib harness, hip strap, shoulder cuff, tray – assist the individual? Remember with these straps they must allow for breathing and be adjustable depending on the type of clothing worn. They must also be easily removable for reasons of safety, for example, quick removal of the individual from the chair if choking.

If using a tray, there are a number of factors which should be considered.

- *Size*. What is the purpose of the tray? The chair must be manoeuvrable through doors, etc.
- *Height*. Is the tray providing support through the person's arms while also being a rest for the communication device, switch, power chair control? The clinician should try the functional activity to ensure the tray height is correct.
- Most trays do not provide sufficient support for electronic communication devices.
- Should the tray be padded? If it is being used for support, or if the individual's arms are likely to get 'caught' on the tray, then this option must be considered. People with involuntary movements can get locked into positions.
- Do bars or trays assist positioning? Bars appear to assist initially but not in the long term. When used with arm splints (elbow extension gaiters) extreme caution is advised as the individual is often locked into extension which cannot be seen under the splints.

When the individual appears seated in the optimum position, the clinician should try functional activities again. The individual should be taken off chair for twenty minutes, checked for any pressure marks (red areas), and then returned to the seat. It is important to consider:

- Can the clinician get the individual into position easily?
- Can the carers get the individual into position easily?

In light of these trials, the clinician should reassess the functional position. Modifications may need to be done now and then during a trial period. Further improvements may be required over time.

The team will need to work with the individual and the carers regarding his ability and need to communicate depending on positions and environment. A checklist of environments and communication needs, opportunities, and positions can be drawn up like the one shown on Table 10.1.

Table 10.1 *Environments & communication needs*

Environment	Place	Equipment	Communication
1 Bathroom	Toilet	Special chair	Signal for assistance
2 Bathroom	Shower	Special chair	
3 Bedroom	Bed	None	Call to be turned

- In situation 1, the individual's ability to hit the switch – for example, a gross swipe – may operate a Bigmack® switch with a message to say 'I'm ready', allowing the individual privacy in the bathroom.
- In situation 2, a laminated communication board can be used by eye pointing so that the individual can request how he wishes to be showered – for example, if he wants his hair washed or not.
- In situation 3, the individual may be able to shout for assistance or may require night-time positioning to facilitate maintaining physical range of movement while also allowing a switch to be positioned and operated to call for assistance.

This process should be followed through for all environments, remembering that equipment is not always the solution.

CHAPTER 11

Early Scanning

Assessment and Training for Visual Scanning

Assessment and training must be ongoing with individuals with severe physical disability. As the skill develops, the complexity of the task can be increased. The ultimate goal is that the skill becomes automatic for the individual so that he can concentrate on the other factors involved in the communication interaction. Discussion with an ophthalmologist of the visual materials to be used in assessment and therapy for the individual can give very valuable information on the individual's visual and visual perception skills.

The following are some areas for discussion.

- At what distance should objects/pictures be placed?
- What is the minimum size, and optimum colour/contrasts of objects/pictures?
- In which field of vision is the best placement of objects/pictures?

This discussion can reduce the amount of trials the clinician may have to use to assess these skills. The clinician can also establish the individual's level of visual function in some other important areas.

The following are guidelines for evaluation:

- Does the individual need to move his head to look at something beyond the midline?

- How far out to the periphery (left/right) can the individual visually attend to an object?
- Can the individual visually track the object from the periphery across the midline to the opposite side without stopping or blinking (horizontally, vertically and diagonally)?
- Can the individual fix his gaze on an object, then shift the gaze to another object, fix on the new one and shift back to the original stimulus or to the midline?
- When presenting activities to an individual it is important to do a task analysis of the skills required in relation to visual scanning and tracking.
- The individual should be placed in a position where he has sufficient support and stability for the head so that the eyes can be used independently.

Tracking games can be used to assess the ability to track from left to right, and right to left. This will allow the clinician to assess at what point on the periphery the object is first picked up in the visual field and whether there are any difficulties in crossing the midline. The following points are of importance when evaluating tracking skills.

- If the individual is in an upright position, the target should be moved horizontally at eye level, for example, a ball can be moved along a track from side to side.
- Depending on the response received, an auditory cue, such as a bell in the ball, may be required and the size and speed can be varied to see which best suits the individual.
- Many individuals with severe disability require very slow movement across the midline and for some, the object needs to stop while the individual blinks and then picks up the object again.
- If the individual is lying supported in a prone position, an activity such as blowing one bubble and catching it on the wand can be used to track across horizontally for the individual.
- It may be found that the individual can visually accommodate the object in his peripheral vision better than in the midline and to one side better than to the other.

- It is important to use this information when asking the individual to visually attend to two objects and perhaps make a choice. The objects must be placed in the individual's optimum field of vision.
- If the individual had difficulty crossing the midline during the tracking game and/or had a difficulty in looking to one side, it would be important to take this into account and perhaps give him more time and cues to shift his gaze from one object to the other.
- Shifting the gaze from one object to a second is known as linear scanning and this can be built upon to include three, four and more objects.
- In assessing for linear scanning, it is important to know how many objects/pictures the individual can scan at one time. It must be first established that the individual can identify the different objects or pictures.
- Initially, the individual may be permitted to eye point to his own choice, for example, non-directed choice.
- It is then important to set up the activity whereby the individual must eye point to directed choices also. Once again, the objects and/or pictures should be at the individual's eye level.
- There is a limit to the number of objects/pictures which can be presented in a linear fashion and an E-Tran frame or a body vest can be used to increase the number of targets, and also the position.
- If all four sides are being used – for example, the four corners – the individual must start circular scanning to make a directed selection.
- The number of targets should not be increased beyond 15, as in circular scanning there is no real beginning or end and it is a difficult organisational task. A note is taken of the number of targets, their size and spacing.
- Simple communication boards are usually laid out so that they can be scanned through a group, then item system.
- Colour coding is often used to assist in the development of language but it also assists the individual to identify the different areas on the board/device more quickly and visually differentiate the areas.
- It would be important to assess how closely the groups can be placed and how closely the individual pictures can be placed within each group.

- The communication board may need to be made up in such a way that each group can be shown separately initially, so as to decrease the amount of distractibility provided by the second or third group. Individuals with visual figure ground perceptual difficulties will benefit from this.
- To assist the communication partner's ability to interpret the selections correctly, she should point to each object or picture, so that the individual can choose the required selection.
- It would be important to take into account the speed at which the pictures or objects are scanned and also the length of time needed for the individual to give the required motor response indicating the choice.
- A common reason for breakdown in the communication process with communication boards is that the communication partner who is scanning the selection set does so too quickly, the individual does not have sufficient time to give the motor response to indicate the choice and as a result, the whole group is scanned unsuccessfully.
- If this process is repeated, both sides may become frustrated.
- The individual who is trying to make the selection may then begin to have difficulties in dealing with the anticipation of the required choice approaching, and may realise that he will be unable to indicate this. This may cause an individual who has high muscle tone or fluctuating tone to become very anxious and therefore the tone will increase. In turn, the individual may lose his position in his chair and become very distressed. It is therefore very important to establish the correct speed of scan for the individual.

CHAPTER 12

Symbol Assessment

Introduction

Symbol assessments can be carried out either utilising symbols in isolation from the communication system, or using symbols set up on communication aids. However, if there are doubts about scanning abilities and access issues, then to improve reliability of results, symbols should be used in isolation. In assessing understanding of symbols, the clinician is wise to apply the concepts of control and connection to activities. For example:

- Making people do things, eg, 'Daddy jump'
- Establishing a social component, and
- Introducing humour.

Blank symbols should be utilised, where appropriate (particularly where any symbols can be selected), to improve reliability of responding and interpretation.

Again, because we need to focus on the potential of individuals as well as their skills, tasks should include teaching (to evaluate if the individual can learn a new task) as well as testing. This is because non-speaking individuals may have limited experience, not because of their ability but because of their reduced activity and probable reduced control of their daily lives leading to passivity and communication-partner dominated 'conversations'.

The speech & language therapist should assess for a number of symbol-related issues. These are:

- *Level of representation:*
  - Objects
  - Miniature objects
  - Photographs
  - Coloured pictures
  - Black-and-white line drawings
  - Words

- *Level of representation within symbol systems*, for example, concreteness/transparency to abstractness.
- *Size of symbols*
- *Number of symbols*
- *Ability to combine symbols*, for example:
  - Semantic compaction
  - Syntactic structures
  - Location
  - Levels

Level of Representation

The clinician should prepare a number of matching triplicate pairs. The stimulus should be based on language levels. For example, if an individual recognises nouns and actions, then stimuli based on a combination of these should be used for this task. Examples of the various levels using this sample are given in Table 12.1.

Please note that there is also a level of abstractness within symbol systems – for example, black-and-white line drawings. An example of this is Bliss®, where symbols are more abstract than, for example, in Picture Communication Symbols® (PCS). If the individual is a candidate for Bliss®, then the individual's understanding of this must be evaluated. For the purpose of the general symbol assessment in this section, one system such as the general PCS® type should be utilised.

There is no need to assess for words in this section if the literacy assessment has already been carried out and literacy levels established. If

Table 12.1 *Examples of symbols at different levels of representation*

Level of Representation	Example
Objects	Doll, ball, book
Miniature objects	Miniatures of the above
Photographs	Photographs of the above
Colour pictures	Colour pictures of the above
Black-and-white line drawings	Line drawings of the above as available in symbol systems
Abstract symbols	Bliss®
Words	Words only of the above

an individual is able to read words, then obviously, setting tasks to evaluate for level of symbol representation is not necessary. To carry out this assessment correctly, labels should not be attached to these symbols at any stage, with the exception of the words levels of representation.

The clinician does not have to complete all the levels of this task. For example, if the clinician feels the individual is capable of reading, then this is the level at which the assessment should start. If the clinician feels black-and-white line drawings will be understood, then there is no need to start trials at the previous levels. Items should be presented at the various levels – for example, all photographs together. The individual is asked to identify the various stimuli through general directions, such as:

'Show me the … '
'Where is the …?'

For individuals who do not understand at initial levels, the clinician should not proceed onto other tasks in this section. It is likely this individual will have therapy needs in language and symbol recognition areas.

Size of Symbols

Where an individual can utilise the smallest of symbols, then the potential for the number of communication messages available to them at one time increases significantly, whether this be on a low-tech system such as a communication board or on a high-tech dynamic device.

Typically, symbol size is dictated by the number of rows and columns in the system layout. The best way to assess the individual's abilities in this area is to utilise ready-made overlays available either commercially or on the Boardmaker® software which is capable of producing overlays of varying numbers and suitable for a number of devices. These can be of various constructions – for example, 2 columns by 2 rows, or a 128 location overlay from static devices. Assessment using ready-made or prepared overlays will speed up the assessment process considerably.

Although the clinician should have a range of stimuli available, it may not be necessary to apply them all during testing as noted previously. We recommend starting at the level (that is, number of symbols) appropriate to the age and/or cognitive functioning of the individual. This will cut the testing time.

If more specific procedures are necessary, the clinician should continue as follows. Symbols should be selected based on the individual's receptive language level to rule out unreliable results. Two sets per size level should be attempted, to ensure validity of the individual's responses to the size stimuli. As the issue is not the number of stimuli (location) an individual can utilise, but the size he can select, these stimuli symbols can be placed apart when presenting them to the individual.

The clinician should have an array of symbols prepared. Recommended sizes are ½-inch (1.2 cm), 1-inch (2.5 cm), 2-inch (5 cm), 4-inch (10 cm), 6-inch (15 cm) and 8-inch (20 cm). However, as low-tech systems are flexible, if an individual is not able to use any size previously mentioned, the clinician could try further enlargements. It is unlikely, however, if the individual cannot recognise any of the symbols at this level, that the symbol size is the issue. For example, if the individual has failed to understand symbols in the previous activity, then this is a problem of symbol recognition, one relating to the symbols presented and not their size. The clinician should present symbols sets based on size. She should present set 1 and direct the individual to:

'Find the ...' or 'Show me the ...'

Number of Symbols – Location Level

Ideally, the clinician should have a number of overlays available at various size levels, which should be used based on the individual's response to the previous task (that is, the size of the symbol). It is not necessary to be exhaustive in this section. For example, if the individual can identify 2 inch (5 cm) symbols, then an array of symbols should be copied onto an A4 size sheet. This should represent the largest number offered. If the individual can identify symbols at this location level, then no further testing of this area is needed. The clinician should present fewer symbols only if the individual is not able to cope with this number. For example, if an individual cannot respond to a block of 8×2 inch (5 cm) squares, try a block of 4×2 inch (5 cm) squares. It is again important to note that, as children develop, so does their capacity for coping with larger numbers of symbols on a page. The clinician should select symbols with which the individual is familiar from previous tasks, based on language levels and level of symbolic representation.

This task can be carried out on devices with predesigned overlays. If the individual is a candidate for a high-tech system, it is preferable to use communication aids to facilitate this part of the assessment process provided scanning and access are not problematic. A number of aids come preprogrammed – for example, Deltatalker® (128 location at ½-inch [1.2 cm] size), Spokesman® (16 location 1-inch [2.5 cm] size). Other devices can carry a number of different sized overlays which can be preprogrammed for ease of testing. Examples of these are the Alphatalker® and Macaw®. In other words, there are communication aids which can be programmed or come preset which will facilitate preparation for this part of the session. These do not have to be used with switch access. Direct access can be used where necessary or row-column questions (eg, 'Is it this row?') by the clinician can be utilised to facilitate the individual. Similarly, overlays can be copied on to paper and used in isolation.

The symbol size impacts on the number of symbols an individual can use, and so with some individuals the number used and therefore the range of symbols available will be naturally reduced. For example, an individual who is able to select at a 4 inch (10 cm) × 4 inch (10 cm) level (or large objects) may only be able to use a limited number of symbols at once, either practically or cognitively. (Practically the clinician needs to think in terms of an E-Tran or communication folder or communication aids which can provide an enlarged symbol size – for example, Cameleon®, Alphatalker®.)

Symbols should ideally be placed side by side as this will probably be the method by which they will be used in practice. However, some individuals require spacing between symbols to facilitate access and scanning (see Chapters 14 and 15). The individual should be asked to identify between four and six symbols on those sets (or the maximum available).

Combining Symbols/Encoding

This section will be divided into a number of main tasks, which are features of a number of communication aids and symbol systems discussed previously.

With some activities, to make them more realistic, the clinician may want to store utterances on voice-output devices or single-channelled voice-output aids such as the Bigmack®. For example, when an individual uses the combination *Level 1 + Symbol 1,* the clinician could press the voice-output device to say 'My name is …'

Semantic Compaction
This can be carried out in the following ways:

- Using photographs/symbols.
- Programming static aids for semantic compaction, such as the Alphatalker®, Macaw® or Eclipse®. This can be done using static aids.
- Using programmes such as Language, Living and Learning®, Unity®, etc, on the Deltatalker®;

The clinician must evaluate not only whether the individual can understand the concept of semantic compaction but also whether the individual can remember a number of semantic compaction selections.

The clinician should select a number of combinations but it is not necessary to cover all types of combinations (that is, associative, categorical, feature-based, etc), as outlined previously. At least five combinations should be selected preferably from ready-made programmes. If photographs are being used, the above rules for combining can apply. For example, the clinician can designate 'Apple' to be a starter icon for fruit.

Therefore *Apple + Moon = Banana,* etc. A jigsaw-type game can prove useful here, for example, show the 'banana' and ask the individual to find the combination from a selected group which produces the target word.

The individual should be taught the rules of semantic compaction by explaining that combinations of symbols can make new meanings and this should be demonstrated. The individual should be taught the selected combinations one at a time and asked to produce them as they are taught. All combinations should be placed in front of the individual and then the individual should be directed to:

'Show me which ones make the word/phrase ...'

In order to thoroughly evaluate this concept, the individual should be advised that a single symbol such as 'Sausage', retains its original meaning and this should be evaluated within the session.

Levels

If the individual has the potential to use a static device with a number of levels, as described previously, the ability to understand this concept of levels, and therefore one symbol having multiple meanings, needs to be probed. However, the clinician must be aware that most of the communication aids with this feature cannot be utilised by the individual unless direct access is used. This can be done on aids like the Blackhawk®, Chatbox® or Portacam®, but if this is not available to the clinician, a symbol code can be taught and then evaluated. See Table 12.2, for example.

Table 12.2 *Levels examples*

Level 1	Symbol 1	My name is ...
Level 2	Symbol 1	I live at ...
Level 3	Symbol 1	My phone number is ...
Level 4	Symbol 1	I use this to communicate ...

The individual should be taught:

- Each button/symbol carries specific information
- The button/symbol that changes levels

- The button/symbol that carries specific information, for example, Icon 1 = identification information.
- The rule that a single button/symbol can carry different utterances if used in combination with the Level button/symbol.

Level buttons can be colour coded to facilitate the individual.

The clinician should select at least two icons, that is, eight messages to teach, one at a time, and arrange the symbols as follows:

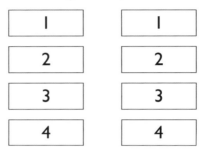

Once taught, the levels should be evaluated to see if they have been learned. The clinician can say:

'Show me how you would say …'

Locators/Indicators

These symbols are used to add meaning to symbols or messages already selected. They are typically redundant in semantic content when used in isolation. For example:

1   The Bliss® *Opposite* locator:

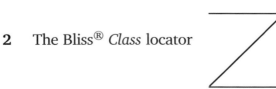

2   The Bliss® *Class* locator

For this activity the clinician should select two to three locators. She will also need a set of noun symbols – for example, 'Apple', 'Happy', 'Big', 'Shirt'. The individual should be taught the rules of combination. First, the single symbol (eg, 'Happy') retains that meaning but that when combined with the *Opposite* Locator, the symbol makes a new word (that is, 'Sad'). With the *Class* Locator the individual can be told that when this is combined with a noun such as 'Shirt', the communication partner will understand the individual is trying to communicate about something in this category. Both rules should be taught but only one at a time.

Once the individual is trained, the clinician can then present the symbols and ask the individual to identify words. For example:

'Show me how you would say "Sad".'
and
'How would you help me understand it was
clothes you are talking about?'

The individual will need to be taught that the words he is expected to make by combining symbols are not available to him by a single symbol themselves. The clinician may say, for example:

'You know sometimes when you want to say something and it is not on your board, well this is like that. It is done by using other pictures to make the word.'

Grammatical and Syntactical Constructions
If this has not been assessed already, it can be evaluated for as outlined in Chapter 13.

Index/Master Pages
Another skill that is worth assessing is the individual's ability to use an index page. This is a feature common to both communication folders and dynamic systems. This page functions like an index of chapters in a book, that is, you check it to find which page to go to for the information you want. It is easy to make one of these with symbols and words, and it may look something like Table 12.3.

Table 12.3 *A sample index page*

Family	Food	Letters
School	People	Numbers
Places	Activities	Football

The clinician should have follow-on pages. That is, if the clinician wants the individual to point to the Food page, then a Food page should appear as the result of the individual touching the same. This will help the individual's understanding of the function and concept and produce more reliable results.

Once the individual understands how to access symbols/messages using a master page, then the clinician should direct him to find specific messages on the individual pages, but using the master page. For example:

'Show me how you would tell somebody you needed to go to the toilet.'

The clinician should conduct a number of trials to assess for reliability in understanding the concept.

Other Expansion Techniques
On some voice-output devices – for example, the Lightwriter® – two keys may contain set phrases which have been stored under codes. For example: the memory key and another key (eg, N for Name) can produce personal identification information such as 'My name is …' Table 12.4 gives a few more possible examples.

Table 12.4 *Memory Key expansion examples*

Memory Key +	A =	I'm going to *America* on holiday.
Memory Key +	B =	Can I have a *Beer* please?
Memory Key +	C =	My *Car* is a ...

For an individual with some ability to recognise letters, this can be a valuable expansion tool. The clinician can use a communication aid such as the Lightwriter® or ready-made symbols (which can be colour coded).

The clinician should teach the rule of combination verbally and by demonstrating with the communication aid. The different combinations should then be taught to the individual. This can then be evaluated by asking:

'Which one says "I live at"?'

or

'How would you say "Can I have a beer please"?'

or

'Can you remember how to say "My car is ..."'

Alpha or numeric encoding is also possible where messages are stored under letters or numbers. They can be stored in a number of ways. Beukelman & Mirenda (1992) give a number of examples, including:

1   Encoding under the initial letters of the message (salient letter encoding). For example:

HH = 'Hello. How are you?'
---

2   Alpha numeric encoding where messages are stored under a letter and number. For example:

G (greeting). 1 (number 1). = 'Hello. How are you?'

Further comments
With all these sections, the clinician should note how easily the individual understood the concept and was able to put it into practice. Examples of comments are:

1   Achieved easily
2   Achieved with some demonstration
3   Needed repeated demonstration, and
4   Not achieved.

With the dynamic communication aids, there are a number of functions which have not been addressed here. These include the ability to move between pages, to clear the bar at the top of the page which produces speech, to use a particular function such as 'Backspace'. There are also particular functions relevant to specific devices. An example is the use of Pop-up Pages on the Dynavox® which lets the individual access, for example, morphological markers. The clinician is best to target these using the actual aids.

If this is not feasible however, then creating simulated functions using symbols is possible. To do this, the clinician needs to understand what the features of particular devices are, what she wants to evaluate in particular, and the significance of the functions. In ideal circumstances, all the above should be carried out utilising the actual devices. This will give the clinician an accurate representation of the individual's ability to cope with all aspects of the device simultaneously. It is also important to obtain the individual's reaction to the visual aspects of the communication aid, such as size, layout, etc.

CHAPTER 13

Language Assessment

Introduction

As with previous forms of assessment, it appears that with language assessment it is best to utilise a combination of:

- Modified standardised instruments
- Parent/carer reporting
- Criterion-referenced tasks, and
- Targeted observation.

The areas targeted are outlined below.

- *Standardised assessments*, modified or adapted to the evaluative potential of language skills with regard to AAC.
- *Language function,* tasks to identify the potential to use a system.
- *Vocabulary levels,* to identify the level and organisation of system.
- *Association skills,* especially those typical of that required on a static device, particularly with regard to semantic compaction abilities.
- *Ability to categorise* objects and list pages, more typical of a dynamic system or communication folder.
- *Ability to formulate grammatical and syntactical constructions,* typical of a communication board and also available on some high-tech systems.

With regard to low-tech systems, the above information is helpful in organising the layout of the communication board.

- *Abstract language skills,* such as figurative speech. The presence of such skills can help a clinician in deciding on the type of symbols to recommend, and the device to be utilised.
- *Literacy skills,* to help evaluate the role literacy will take in a system.

Assessment Guidelines

The chapter on symbols more fully explores symbol characteristics; however, for the purpose of this chapter, pictures or symbols can be interchanged depending on the individual except where stated otherwise. Communication aids can also be set up for tasks. However, the clinician should feel comfortable about language and symbol levels if taking this route. For example, if the individual has apparent issues around access or switching and scanning, it may be wiser to utilise photographs/symbols in isolation first to ensure reliability of results and so that there is minimal confusion about which skills are impacting on the use of a device. Software such as the Boardmaker® can facilitate in this by producing a number of ready-made overlays (see Appendix).

The tasks/activities outlined on the following pages are intended to sample communication skills rather than to be a complete representation of a person's abilities.

Language Functions

As the focus of these tasks is communication and not symbolic ability, the clinician can use either objects or pictures/symbols. For the sake of brevity, not all options are mentioned in each section. The use of symbol level should depend on the potential of the user. For example, if the individual is severely cognitively impaired, objects would be appropriate. If the individual is felt to be relatively competent, then pictures should be used. In this section, for example, the clinician, by using pictures, will obtain an idea of not only the individual's ability regarding language functions, but also about the use of symbols to achieve communication. Please remember, however, in this section the primary focus needs to be on communication and reliability of results.

Task 1: Single Request/Communication Intent/Cause & Effect

1   Have picture (or just bottle) of bubbles.
2   Place in front of individual as appropriate – for example, on tray, held upright, using E-tran.
3   Hold actual object (bubbles) in hand and say:

'These are bubbles (*show*); this is a picture of bubbles (*point to picture*). When you want me to blow the bubbles, look at (*touch*) the bubbles (*picture*) and I will blow the bubbles'

---

4   Do a trial run. Be specific in your requests. For example:

'Look at the picture now. Good, you looked at the picture; now I will blow the bubbles'.

---

5   Advise the individual that you will blow the bubbles when he looks at the picture/bubbles. Do so immediately when he does to reinforce his communication.

Alternatives
- 'More' (To request more of anything)
- 'Car' (Roll car along the table)
- 'Video' (Turn on and off)
- 'Funny face' (Make funny faces)
- 'Chocolate' (To request chocolate)
- 'Dog' (To request battery-operated dog)
- 'Jump' (to request a person jumps up and down).

Task 2: Choice Making/Decision Making

1   Have pictures of objects which represent desired/motivating objects or activities, such as bubbles and a balloon.
2   Present the symbols one at a time, labelling them and matching them to the objects as presented.
3   Place appropriately while putting enough space between the symbols so that the individual's response can be reliably interpreted. With some individuals this will need to be at right and left extremes of the individual's body.

4   Do a trial run by demonstrating the task.
5   Ask the individual which object he would like. Tell him to look at the picture of his choice, then reinforce the communication behaviour with the desired object or activity.
6   Repeat.

Alternatives
Use a combination of liked and disliked activities – for example, sweets and book.

Task 3: Control/Initiation + Termination/Decision Making
1   Have video recorder and selection of video tapes. Have pictures or single-channel voice-output switch such as the Bigmack® representing:

'Turn it on.'
or
'A different one, please.'

---

2   Identify objects, explain task and demonstrate pictures. For example:

'When you look at (or touch) this symbol, I will turn the video on. Just like this, OK?'
and
'When you look at (or touch) this symbol, I will change the video and put another one in.'

---

3   Place the pictures, as appropriate. Wait until individual selects 'Turn it on' to start the tape.
4   You may need to deliberately sabotage this by stopping the tape if the individual gets too engrossed in the activity!
5   Repeat.

Alternatives
- Tape recorder and musical tapes
- Switch and battery-operated toys
- 'Stop' instead of or in addition to 'A different one please'. Facilitate this by putting a disliked tape in deliberately and demonstrating:

'Oh, I put the wrong one in. If you want me to stop it, look at the "stop" picture.'

Task 4: Attention/Sequencing

1 Have Mr Potato Head® or cardboard body cutout with parts to attach.
2 Have pictures representing the different body parts and accessories – for example, leg or hat, or use the actual parts (that is, for Mr Potato Head®).
3 Explain the activity. For example:

'When you ask us to put an arm on Mr Potato Head, we will, but first you must tell us what you want to put on him. You can tell me by looking at the picture (*or body part*).'

4 Demonstrate the activity.
5 Repeat.

Alternatives
- Doll and clothes
- Shop set up with selection of items.
- You can select a limited number of body parts and corresponding pictures if you feel the individual cannot cope with too large a selection, just introducing extras as the individual selects.

Task 5: Turn Taking/Directing

1 Have skittles and ball.
2 Have pictures for '*My turn*' and '*Your turn*' (with different faces). A non-symbolic level would be for the individual to look at the appropriate person when it is his turn (there would have to be two other individuals, photographs could also be used).
3 Demonstrate. For example,

'When you point to "Your turn" (or look at me), I will throw the ball at the skittles like this. When you point to "My turn", I will help you throw the ball at the skittles.'

4 Do activity.

Alternatives
- Blocks of varied colour (individual and therapist can take turns selecting colours of blocks to build a tower).
- Dressing a doll.
- Operating a cause-effect toy by switch, if necessary.

Vocabulary Skills
The clinician can use objects, photographs or commercially available sets such as ColorCards™ for the tasks outlined in this section.

Task 6: Basic Vocabulary
The clinician needs to initially establish if the individual has a level of basic vocabulary prior to proceeding with tasks which require more complex semantic skills. This ideally should be done using a vocabulary test with modifications to materials or procedures as outlined previously. However, if this has not yet been carried out or if the individual is severely cognitively/linguistically impaired to render standardised instruments unfeasible, a simple receptive vocabulary check can be carried out to evaluate for this necessary skill.

1 The amount of vocabulary an individual can select is not at issue here but sufficient choices should be administered to ensure an overview of skills. Vocabulary of common items is satisfactory for this purpose.
2 Give the individual a choice of between two and four cards and ask:

'Show me the ...'

3 Ask the individual to identify at least 20 pictures in this way.
4 Again, we focus on potential for learning. If an individual has failed any items, select one initially to teach and repeat some elements of the exercise, this time including the learned vocabulary items.

Continuing Development
- Action words – for example, 'Show me eating', 'Which one is jumping?', etc.
- Adjectives – for example, 'big', 'wet', etc.

Task 7: Association

Same concept

1 Have duplicate sets of objects or photographs, two to three sets are usually sufficient to establish reliability of the concept.
2 Present three photographs/objects, two of which should be matching and one of which is the foil (not a match).
3 Each sequence should be presented in a different order. For example:

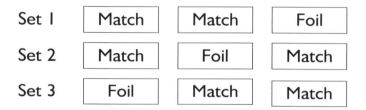

Set 1	Match	Match	Foil
Set 2	Match	Foil	Match
Set 3	Foil	Match	Match

4 Demonstrate the task by pointing at one of the matched pair and saying:

> 'This is a ... Show me one that's the same as this one.'
>
> or
>
> 'Show me the two pictures which are the same.'

5 Repeat.

Continuing Development

- *Similar/alike/go together*
  Organise this activity as the previous one, except the pictures should not be an exact match but have similarities. There are a number of levels within this area. For example:
  1 Very close similarities, eg, short pants and trousers.
  2 Close similarities, eg, pen and paper.
  3 Category similarities, eg, banana and ice cream.

- *Opposite/different from*
  The alternatives need to be very clear. For example, if the opposite pair *'big'* and *'small'* needs to be elicited, the clinician should ideally use:
  1   Big + Big = small
  2   Similar big pictures
  3   Similar objects.

- *Functions*
  Organise this activity as for the basic vocabulary activity. For example, from an array of 'book', 'shirt' and 'pencil', ask:

'Which one do you wear?' 'Show me the one you write with.'
'Which one do we read?'

- *Characteristics*
  Organise this activity as for the basic vocabulary activity and use questions which focus on the features of the items. For example, from an array of 'sun', 'orange' and 'rainbow', ask:

'Which one is hot?' 'Show me the one which has lots of colours.'
'Which one is juicy?'

Task 8: Categorisation

Similar categories
1   The clinician should have a range of objects/photographs from a number of categories – for example, food, clothes, animals, etc.
2   Items should be presented randomly as in the association task with one foil. For example:

banana	dress	apple
dress	hat	book
magazine	apple	book
elephant	table	cat
wheelchair	chair	banana

Any item from another category can be used as a foil.

3   The clinician should proceed as with other sections, this time giving directions such as:

'Show me which ones are food (you can eat).'
'Show me which ones are animals.'

Continuing development
- Develop the level of complexity within categories if appropriate. For example:

  Animals → farm animals, wild animals

  Clothes → winter clothes, outdoor clothes.

Task 9: Compound Words (Analysing Language)
For static devices with the feature of semantic compaction and symbol systems which make new meanings by combining icons, an individual must be able to grasp the idea that symbols can be combined to make other words. Although the concept is analysed more completely in Chapter 12, in this activity we need to obtain an idea of a person's ability to analyse words.

1   Select around five compound words (separated halves which are words in themselves but when combined, can form a new word). For example:
- lighthouse (light and house)
- matchbox (match and box)
- postbox (post and box)
- toothbrush (tooth and brush)
- underwear (under and wear)
- hotdog (hot and dog)

2   Have symbols for each compound word and its separate halves. For example:

| Lighthouse | Light | House |

3   Demonstrate the concept using one set of symbols, such as matchbox. Say:

'I have two pictures here. This is "Match". This is "Box". " Match" and "Box". They are two different words. But if I put them together. Listen. "Matchbox". They make a new word (*show symbol of matchbox*). The two words "Match" and "Box" can make a new word when they are joined.'

---

4   Ask the individual to find compound words. Present three options, for example, lighthouse, underwear, toothbrush.

5   Show the separated pair, for example, 'light' and 'house'. Ask:

'When we put these two words together, which new one do we make?'

Initially, you should just point and see if the individual is able to retrieve this information himself. If not, then you can opt to say the names.

Task 10: Multiple Meanings
Some words and symbols in AAC systems are abstract in nature and have multiple meanings. To utilise these more complex systems, an ability to understand complex language such as multiple meanings and figurative language is a desirable (but not essential) skill. For example, on the LLL® programme from Liberator, the pronoun *I* is represented by the symbol of an eye.

1   Present the two alternatives for a number of sets. For example:
   • *Hand* of the body and the *hand* of a clock
   • *Eye* of the body and *I* as in pronoun
   • *Which* as in question and *witch*

2   Give examples of sentences which can contain the target words and ask the individual to select the appropriate picture for the sentence. For example:

'This one is a question.' 'This one rides on a broomstick.'

and

'The witch wears a pointed hat.' 'Which is your favourite?'

Task 11: Figurative Speech

1   Give examples of figurative speech one at a time, for example, 'A rolling stone gathers no moss'.

2   Provide picture alternatives: one literal and one accurate (that is, representing the true meaning of the saying). Present also a foil (inappropriate) picture. This should ideally be linguistically near the meaning.

3   Ask the individual to identify the accurate picture. For example:

'Listen to this. Show me the pictures which this sentence fits.'

Syntax and Grammar

In this part of the assessment process, we only focus on the very basic constructions to evaluate skills as a significant amount of time could be spent on this area alone.

Task 12: Vocabulary

1   Have a range of symbols for the following:
   - Subjects, for example, He (boy), She (girl), Your (pointing out), My (pointing in).
   - Verbs, for example, kick, swim.
   - Conjunctions, for example, and.

2   The understanding of these words should be checked as with previous activities and previous section. Present the pictures for each group and ask the individual to identify the appropriate picture. For example:

'Show me *He*.'

or

'Show me *She*.'

and

'What a lovely jumper you are wearing. Is that my jumper or yours?
Show me with the pictures.'

Task 13: Construction

The idea of this section is to evaluate whether the individual can combine words to make sentences. This should be assessed for two-word constructions (Subject + Verb, eg, 'Girl kick') and three-word combinations (Subject + Verb + Object, eg, 'Girl kick ball'). The clinician can extend this further, for example, by using adjectives to make four-word constructions (eg, Subject + Verb + Adjective + Object) if felt appropriate. However, the main idea is to formulate an opinion about whether the individual understands the idea of combining words to make sentences.

1   Select two to three photograph/symbol alternatives for each grouping. For example;
    • Subjects – mummy, girl, boy.
    • Verbs – kick, eat, break (ideally these should be action oriented and need a following object to explain the communication fully).
    • Objects – book, plate, chocolate.

2   The clinician should offer the standard phrases such as 'Mummy ate chocolate' and silly alternatives such as 'Mummy ate the plate'.

3   The activity should be demonstrated first and the appropriate sequence placed in front of the individual. For example:

Girl	Kicked	Ball

The activity is demonstrated and the sequence pointed out using clear and simple language (appropriate to the individual's language level and chronological age). For example:

'What did Mummy do? Mummy (*point to picture*) kicked (*point to picture*) the ball (*point to picture*).'

This activity should be commenced at a two-word level and then a three-word level should be targeted if the individual has succeeded at the previous level.

4   Both silly and appropriate activities should be carried out for each group. Once one action is carried out, the individual should be offered a choice of two alternatives for each group. For example, mummy/girl, kick/jump, and plate/ball. One of each should be correct. The clinician can say:

'Watch what happens. See?'
and
'Now you tell me what happened.'

or if probing is necessary:

'Who ate the chocolate?'
'What did she do?'
'What did she eat?'

Continuing Development
● Spontaneous expression can also be targeted in this activity. For example, the individual can tell others what to do given a choice of symbols.
● Adjectives.
● Picture description.

Task 14: Grammatical Understanding
Again a few basic constructions only are targeted in this activity.

1   Select pictures to represent the following morphological markers and a selection of nouns:
    ● Verb + *ing* (jump, dance, laugh, -ing)
    ● Verb + *ed* (jump, dance, laugh, -ed)

2   Demonstrate first. Ask a person in the room, for example, to jump. This person should continue jumping while the task is ongoing.

3   Present the symbols.

Jump	Dance	ing

4   Say

_____
'What is she doing?'
_____

Point to the appropriate combination of pictures emphasising the one which represents the *ing* marker and say:

_____
'She is jump (*point to symbol*) + ing (*point to symbol*). Jumping. When these two pictures go together they make the right word. You show me the next time.'
_____

5   Repeat and present another alternative.

Continuing Development
• To further evaluate more complicated understanding an irregular verb such as *run/ran* can be used.
• The same can be applied for the marker 'ed', but of course the activity should have stopped when the question 'What did she do?' is asked.

Literacy
Standardised literacy assessments can be utilised by modifying them or by using an alphabet board. We tend to use a number of samples rather than administer complete assessments, and select vocabulary at various levels equivalent to various age levels with the individual's age or cognitive ability represented as the median.

   Skills assessed include:

• Letter and number recognition
• Basic (first) reading vocabulary
• Intermediate vocabulary which would equate to a midway point between the first words and an individual's age, and

- Age-equivalent vocabulary.
- Additionally, sentence reading which is evaluated by providing one sentence and four possible alternatives.

This is only a very basic screening and by no means should be considered a reliable evaluation of reading skills. If an individual displays good skills on these criterion-referenced tasks, then we proceed to standardised assessment of reading and spelling using an alphabet board for the spelling component. Modifications to standardised procedures for physically disabled individuals are usually necessary and this may occur by modifying the stimulus (for example, enlarging the picture stimuli) or adapting the access, for example, by the clinician scanning for the individual, or by offering the individual a choice such as:

Is it 1, 2, 3, or 4?'
---

and by accepting 'Yes' and 'No' signals.

Task 15: Letter and Number Recognition
1   Use an alphabet (or number) board and scanning or direct access, whichever is suitable to the individual's access method.
2   Select a number of consonants, vowels and numbers to test.
3   Ask the individual to identify these on the alphabet (number) board by row-column scanning if appropriate.

Task 16: Vocabulary
1   Select basic, intermediate and age-equivalent vocabulary from a reading test.
2   Provide near (looks like or sounds like) alternatives in addition to an obvious non-alternative. For example, for the word 'Book', the options might be:

boot	book
chair	look

Continuing Development

Sentence recognition can also be approached in the same way. For example, for the sentence 'She kicked the ball', possible alternatives may be:

- He kicked the ball.
- She kicked the ball.
- She kicked the bat.

The individual should be presented with the written sentence first and then the picture alternatives without the written text.

Task 17: Spelling

The individual should be asked to spell using an alphabet board (or a communication aid if he already is familiar with its operation).

1   Familiar words, for example, 'mummy', own name, etc.
2   Words selected as basic words, intermediate words and age-equivalent words as outlined above.
3   Part spell. Confirm the individual does not already know how to spell the word. Ask the individual to find the first letter of the word then the second, and so on. See how far the individual can proceed. Select words beginning with voiced parts initially – for example, 'bee', 'goat'. If appropriate, the clinician can proceed to unvoiced initial consonants and words beginning with vowels. The idea is to see if the individual can analyse words. The clinician may need to exaggerate initial sounds to facilitate the individual in this section.
4   Learned spelling. Select words at levels at which the individual has so far succeeded. Teach the individual how to spell the word by sounding it out and using the alphabet board. The clinician may need to repeat this exercise for an individual word. Then ask the individual to spell it.

CHAPTER 14

Access

Switch Assessment

Please note that there is a difference between switches that are communication aids, for example the single-channelled voice-output switch, the Bigmack®, and switches that are used to access communication aids.

A switch such as the Jelly Bean® switch is useful for assessment as it has a mounting plate which is a little larger than the switch. The clinician, without interfering with the switch, can hold the plate and be confident that it is the individual who activated the switch.

Trialling Switch Use

The clinician should position the individual on the floor and support him with her own body to feel immediately in what positions the individual can successfully initiate a movement. She will also note when the individual is experiencing difficulty – for example, the stimulus is too loud and the individual startles; or the movement required is too difficult and the individual is pushing into extension with spasm.

The clinician should attach the switch to a switch-operated toy such as a barking dog (sound or movement response). The effect should be strong – for example, the toy should move, or part of the toy such as the tail on an animal should move. If the toy has sound, it should not be too loud or sudden as this can elicit a startle response and may frighten the individual. Place the toy so that the individual can see it when it is operated by the switch. With some individuals, the clinician can move directly on to connecting the switch to a voice-output communication aid. This ideally should be a simple one, such as the Bigmack®, initially. However, some individuals can progress quite quickly on to using switches attached to communication aids, and all the skills this requires.

The clinician should hold the switch so that the individual can hit it. She can quickly remove the switch if the individual is inclined to stay on it, or keep hitting it, or become stuck. This reduces the frustration of an incorrect response and prevents the individual from being injured by the switch, or a rigid mounting system. A latching box with timer should be used between the switch and the toy, so that the switch action is on/off and does not need to be held down continuously. By using a timer the individual does not associate the clinician with the toy. When the toy stops, it is important to observe if the individual learns that he has the control to turn it on. There may be a second movement available, which allows two-switch scanning.

Switch Use and Access
The clinician should first assess the hand function for access. Direct access to a toy – for example, pressing a play button on a tape recorder, is the quickest method. Unfortunately many individuals with physical disability who require an AAC system do not have adequate hand function for switch use.

We see a number of individuals referred to us who have been using an extended arm with fisted hand to hit the switch. This method has its drawbacks:

- Usually the effort required is high.
- It can take a long time to achieve the movement.
- The movement is often inaccurate.
- The hand may remain stuck on the switch.

The individual needs to be able to hit the switch without having to look at it. When assessing the switch placement and most accurate repeatable, body movement with the least amount of effort, the clinician should try each body part a number of times while holding the switch in a consistent position for each body part.

While assessing for one control site, it is important to remember the abilities required for step scanning and direct scanning. Switches should be used which have the option of an auditory feedback. The clinician should record what position the individual is in, for example, lying supine on a wedge; in a corner seat with high back to include head, with hip strap, chest strap, and arms placed on table at mid-chest height. She should observe and record how the rest of the body is stabilised. Does the body remain symmetrical for the initiation, action and termination of the movement? Any associated reactions should be recorded. The clinician should record whether auditory feedback is an advantage.

Switch Access Checklist
Use the checklist (Sample Form 12) to record the individual's ability to use different body parts for accessing the switch.

Mounting a Switch
The decision to establish whether the switch can be mounted or not depends on the results of the switch access assessment. It is preferable to trial the switch using a temporary mount or one which will move out of the way if the individual has strong involuntary or strong extensor or flexor spasms. The clinician should use the following procedure:

- Initially repeat the use of the most useful movement found in the switch access assessment while continuing to hold the switch.
- Observe for, and note how quickly the accuracy or efficiency decreases.
- Note whether the switch use causes an increase or decrease in tone or spasms.
- Note if the individual becomes stuck on the switch.

If the individual is experiencing difficulty by becoming caught on the switch, he is not ready to have it mounted. If the individual is achieving some success but is not fully safe, the switch can be mounted using velcro (remember: hook velcro on switch, loop velcro on the chair), or a

147

Switch Access Checklist

Name _____ Date _____

	Movement achieved	Repeated	Reliable	Accurate	Number achieved	Number of opportunities	No. of minutes to fatigue	Efficient
Hand L								
R								
Arm L								
R								
Foot L								
R								
Knee L								
R								
Head L								
R								
Face L								
R								
Chin L								
R								

Signed _____

Sample Form 12 *Switch access checklist*

gooseneck mounting system. A soft switch or wobble leaf switch is also useful at this stage. The temporary mount should be trialled with supervision. Modifications may be necessary for the location of, or the type/size of the switch.

When the individual is using the switch confidently, a permanent rigid mount can be fitted. The Daessy Stem System® is very useful when assessing for a switch mount, as it is very versatile and allows a great many alternative positions to be tried.

Mounting the Device

The communication aid being used in the assessment and trial period must also be mounted. The position of the device will be determined by the requirements of:

- Method of access
- Visual ability, and
- Seating position.

The mounting system should be assessed for its:

- Suitability to safely hold the device
- Compatible mounting block for the wheelchair frame
- Ability to allow the device to be correctly placed for the individual
- Ease of removal to allow the individual in and out of the chair, and
- Aesthetic acceptability to the individual.

CHAPTER 15

Scanning for Communication Systems

Visual Scanning and Direct Selection

When an individual can select the desired object, picture or icon by pointing to it on a communication board, or by pressing an icon on a static communication device or an area of a touch screen on a dynamic device, the individual is said to be making his choice by direct selection. The individual must be able to visually scan all of the targets on the communication system and find the desired choice.

On a static display, such as a communication board or voice-output device, the individual must be able to remember where the different pictures are, if he is to become an efficient and speedy user.

A dynamic display with changing screens is more complex as it requires an individual to constantly adapt and accommodate to the changing visual format, and the different selection sets presented on the display. If the individual cannot remember the position of the different targets, the scanning process is extremely slow. The individual will have to scan each row, picture by picture, line by line until he finds the required one.

Visual Scanning and Indirect Selection

If the individual cannot use direct selection to access the communication device, then an indirect scanning system must be utilised. With indirect selection there are intermediary steps which must be taken to select the message. When using a communication board, the scanning is done by the communication partner. The scanning is controlled by a switch on a communication device. The individual must be able to visually track the alternate selections while also scanning to the desired choice. The switch activation must become automatic so that the individual can attend to the communication device and the communication interaction.

When looking at a communication system which is operated by indirect selection the speed of the scanning is very important, as is the layout and format of the scanning. The communication aid must give feedback to the individual regarding which item is ready for selection. This is given in different ways by different devices either by LED lights, or shading or colour changes. The individual must be able to see the changes to operate the system.

There are a number of different ways in which communication aids can operate the scanning (see Figure 15.1) and many communication systems offer more than one variation. When deciding on a communication device it is important to establish which particular method of scanning best suits the individual.

The clinician should review the information obtained regarding visual and visual perceptual skills, and correct positioning of the individual. Switch use, accuracy and timing should also be reconsidered.

- Where should the device be located? Does the individual have better peripheral or control vision?
- Can the individual cross the midline? Should the device be placed off centre?
- Does the individual lose position if he has to look up or down?
- How wide is the individual's range of vision?
- How far apart were pictures spaced?
- Can he identify line drawings?
- How many pictures can he scan at a time and what detail can he cope with within a picture?

The individual who has had experience using a switch may be accurate but slow, when the timing is not important to the process such as when operating a toy through a switch and timing box. The process of using a single switch on a communication device is more complex. There are three ways that the process can operate any of the scanning sets.

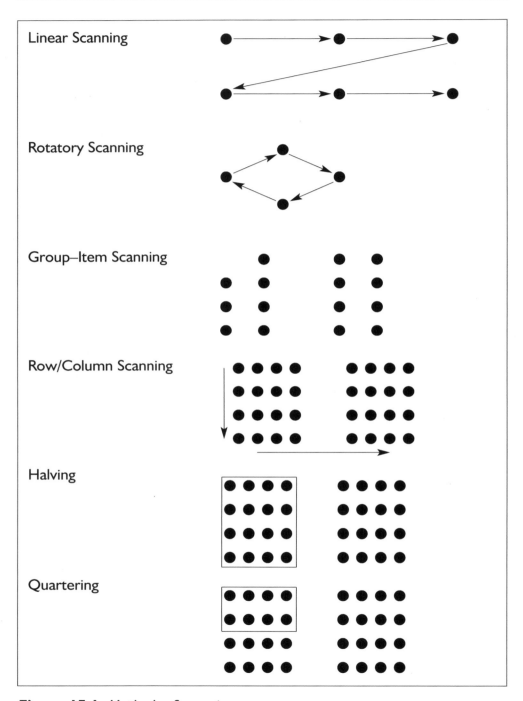

Figure 15.1 *Methods of scanning*

- *Automatic scanning.* The individual starts the scanning by hitting a single switch and the targets are highlighted one by one at a pre-set speed, and remain on the target for a pre-set duration. The switch must be activated again when the desired target is highlighted. This requires the ability to wait for the desired target and to activate the switch quickly and accurately.
- *Step scanning.* This can be achieved in two ways:
  1 Activating the switch to move from one target to the next, one step at a time. When the desired target is reached the second switch may be activated to select it.
  2 Activating the switch one step at a time as in (1) and then making a selection by waiting (no activation) for a pre-set specified length of time.

  The process described in (1) requires the ability to use one switch very accurately and constantly while also being able to activate a second switch less often. The process described in (2) also requires the ability to activate one switch consistently while also being able to stop and wait with accuracy. Step scanning can be very fatiguing.
- *Inverse scanning.* The switch must be held closed/activated until the desired target is reached. The switch must then be released and this makes the selection. This is also a fatiguing method and requires a high level of motor control and attention.

For assessment purposes the automatic method should be tried first.

Many computer programmes have very clear scanning cues and built-in levels of complexity which facilitate assessment. The clinician should consider the following:

- Limiting the number of options for selection, especially for young children and first-time users with severe disability.
- Setting a slow scanning speed and where possible a long acceptance time.
- Starting with linear scanning with two pictures, she should note the individual's ability to activate the switch accurately while keeping

sessions short. If difficulties arise, the causes should be noted. For example:

- ◆ Change (increase) in tone while waiting, (anticipation)
- ◆ Double hitting switch
- ◆ Hitting switch and inability to release it
- ◆ Activating switch just after desired selection, and
- ◆ Any other difficulties.

Initially the individual may need time to familiarise himself with the system, and to understand the timing and that the opportunity will arise again. The clinician should:

- Adjust the speed up/down
- Ensure that the switch is in the correct position, and
- Ensure switch position is not encouraging abnormal pattern of movement.

Individuals who have severe movement disorders such as cerebral palsy, will require many training/assessment sessions at different levels using different methods to facilitate effective use of a single switch for a communication device. Clinicians should consider:

- Computer programmes designed for single-switch use
- Rotary scanners with person-specific themes
- Limited selections on communication device.

As accuracy improves, the number of targets and speed of scanning can be increased. Trials can be made for the most efficient scanning set for the individual.

CHAPTER 16

Voice-Output Communication

The easiest method of matching an individual with a communication aid is to let the individual try out a range of devices. Only at this stage can the individual, carer and clinicians make an informed choice.

Introduction

Recently, there has been a move towards use of the term 'speech-output communication aids' (SOCAs) in place of the long used term 'voice-output communication aids' (VOCAs). As the latter is more commonly recognised, and it also reflects the personal implications of AAC use (as some of our adult clients say 'It [the communication aid] gave me a voice…'), we will use the term VOCA.

Of course, the essential skill for the clinician in this case is a comprehensive understanding of both individual devices and their advantages and disadvantages, in addition to a comprehensive knowledge of the range of devices on the market. The range of VOCAs on the market is large and growing. The obvious bonus of this is the benefit to users and potential users. The downside may be a tendency towards confusion and indecision for the clinician, individual and carers, and a potential for focusing on the technology in the decision-making process and not the individual. The question the clinician should ask when considering a high-tech system is:

'How do we match the user with a voice-output device?'

The simple answer is:

1. Analyse all the information gained from the assessment process thus far.
2. Trial the individual on voice-output devices based on the individual's levels as identified during the assessment process, and
3. If necessary, provide a communication aid for a diagnostic period.

This stage of the process is required for the following reasons:

- For the clinician to identify the individual's specific response to and use of aids including the individual's ability to integrate all his skills when using a communication aid. The clinician will be able to identify potential problems.
- For the individual and carer to see the actual devices and range of devices, and their specific characteristics.
- For the individual to have 'hands-on' experience with devices and determine his own feelings about them. It is at this stage that the clinician will often see the user or carers express decided preferences for one type of VOCA or one specific aid.

With some individuals it is possible to bypass some of the previous sections or activities and proceed straight to trialling them on voice-output systems. These individuals usually adapt quickly to using a communication aid. However, the range available must still be considered and the clinician may need to administer parts of sections outlined previously.

Limiting the Options
At this stage the clinician will have a good idea of the individual's skills and problem areas and should be able to limit the options available to the individual. For example:

- If an individual needs switches to access a device, then systems which do not have this feature will obviously not be of use. For example, the Blackhawk® at time of writing only has direct-access options, and therefore indirect access and scanning are not available to users who need them.

- An individual who can use direct access only with the help of a keyguard, for example, will not be able to use a device without this feature. If the aid has this facility, is one available with the appropriate symbol number and size? Some devices come with a range of overlays – for example, 8 location, 32 location, etc. Others may only have one and this may not suit the individual's needs.

- Does the individual need a communication aid which will be portable? If so, what is available and is it light enough to facilitate an individual with a physical disability?

- Does the individual need a device with other functions - for example, environmental controls, a word processor? Some devices like the Cameleon® are PCs with communication programmes, others like the Deltatalker® can link to computers.

- An individual who requires enlarged symbols will probably not benefit from a portable device which, by the very nature of its size, usually has smaller symbols. (However, some dynamic devices now have a magnifying facility.) Those with adaptable overlays or number of symbols are likely to be less useful because of the limited number of symbols that will then be available to the individual.

- If an individual shows no ability to understand semantic compaction, then communication aids which are organised around this feature may not be part of the assessment process.

- If an individual has a specific need – for example, to communicate only a limited number of messages – then devices which are more linguistically and technologically complex would be of little benefit and certainly not an effective use of monetary resources.

- Evaluation of AAC is not limited to the external or internal features of the device. It must include thorough evaluation of the software contained within the aid. Consideration of the software packages on the device can significantly affect prescription. For example, the Dynavox® range has software which is linguistically more complex than some of its dynamic cousins. The Cameleon® has both Talking Screens® and the literacy-based EZKeys® package. The features of these individual software packages are integral to the individual-device match.

The clinician should therefore select potential devices for this part of the evaluation based on the individuals needs and skills.

Some features on communication aids can be flexible, and therefore the device can be adapted to the needs of the individual. For example:

- Static systems such as Alphatalkers® and Macaws® can be set up with different numbers of symbols (overlays). Dynamic systems function similarly.
- Some devices, such as those mentioned above, have capacity for both single-icon selection and semantic compaction.

Preparing the Communication Aid

A little preparation often goes a long way for this part of the process. Devices can be set up with a variety of personal information that relates to the individual. For example, devices can be set up with:

- *Identification information*, such as the:
  - ◆ Name of the individual.
  - ◆ Family names.
  - ◆ Friends' names.
  - ◆ Favourite and least favoured school activities.
  - ◆ Regular favoured pastimes, etc.

- *Connecting phrases*, such as:

  'That's silly.'
  'Daddy always burns the toast.'
  or
  'That's a load of rubbish.'

- Phrases accompanying *social routines*, such as:

  'Hello.' 'Lovely day.'
  or
  'Goodbye.'

- Symbols that facilitate *choice making*.
- *Jokes* appropriate to the level of understanding of the individual.
- *Motivational phrases*, such as:

'I love (*name*) football team.'

or

'I love (*name*) television programme.'

- *Motivational pages*, such as a fast food page from a favourite restaurant, a McDonald's page, for example.

When trialling the devices, particular features may need to be altered or introduced, based on the individual's needs and performance during assessment. These include:

- The *scanning speed.*
- The *type of scanning* available – for example, auditory and visual scanning.
- The ability to use *functions particular to the communication aid,* such as the *Page Link* (to get from one page to another on category-based systems), *Clear* buttons to clear the bar on the screen, and the *Speak Display* icon which will let the individual 'speak' a complete sentence that he has produced.
- Use of other features on devices such as the *spell mode.*
- The *voice type* on the communication aid where feasible.
- *The screen* and the individual's ability to 'read' it.

The clinician must also take into account information already gathered during the assessment process and how it is applied to the use of a voice-output device. For example:

- Is the individual able to utilise symbols on a communication aid? What are the most appropriate settings regarding the number, spacing and size of these symbols?
- Does a visual impairment necessitate specific device requirements?
- What are the individual's requirements regarding access and the accuracy of switch use?

- If the device is to be mounted, how is this to be done and what are the specific requirements around this?

In the very recent past, Voice Output Software has emerged onto the AAC scene and has the potential to be used on a laptop computer for some individuals. Given that it is in the very early stages of development at the time of writing, it will not be commented on further here, but clinicians should consider its potential for individuals.

Demonstration

It is up to the clinician to demonstrate precisely how the devices/software are used and then give the individual opportunities to practise. It is always a good policy to explain each device in detail to the individual and carers. This includes:

- Details of the operation of the aid
- Its advantages and disadvantages generally
- Its advantages and disadvantages relative to the individual's skills and needs, and
- Accurate responses to any questions the individual, carers or other clinicians may have.

Trialling the Communication Aids

The clinician should then try out the devices with the individual. It is only really once the individual gets a chance to use and see the different communication aids that he develops a preference, and that the clinician can see how all the features assessed thus far come together on specific communication aids.

We recommend use of Musselwhite & St Louis' (1988) principles to help in evaluating the potential effectiveness of an AAC system. These can be outlined as:

1 *Accuracy*. How accurate is the individual when using the device?
2 *Speed*. This can be evaluated generally but also specifically. For example, the clinician can choose a number of words on two devices

which may be suitable for the individual, demonstrate them and then ask him to select each of them on each device. The two devices should be presented in random order to rule out learning. Usually five words will give the clinician an idea of the user's potential with each device relative to speed of use.

3   *Effort*. Does the device or certain devices increase the effort required to communicate and will this affect the potential to use the device?

4   *Cognitive demands*. How does the individual cope with the system (dynamic versus static) or means of organising the language (semantic compaction versus categorisational)? How many icons facilitate use of the system?

5   *Listener demands*. Is the primary user and local service provider able to 'understand' the device? Do they wait for and respond to the user's productions?

We would add a sixth separate section to facilitate analysis. This is:

6   *Listener and user attitude towards the device*. This is usually a factor which influences the outcome to a significant degree.

Using the Information Obtained

The clinician should revisit the AAC Needs Profile (Sample Form 4) which was filled out prior to the start of the assessment, and recheck it against the information retrieved from the assessment process.

The clinician's role is to consider all the information obtained and ask general questions to determine which device, if any, best meets the individual needs. The questions which must be asked at this stage are:

• Would this individual benefit from a high-tech device?
• Does the individual want a communication aid?
• Is there one overriding factor (eg, access) which dominates the decision making at this stage?
• Given all factors, what best meets the individual's needs currently?
• If the individual has potential for development, will this device facilitate that development and how does this impact on decision making?

- Are modifications necessary to any part of the system?
- Are there issues around responsibility for the aid which affect the decision making? For example, will the person responsible be able to programme and update the aid, if necessary? In this case, the clinician needs to ask questions such as:
  - ◆ Who will do the programming?
  - ◆ Do they feel comfortable with technology?
  - ◆ Do they understand the time commitment this involves and are they willing to undertake this?

- Finally, when a decision is made to carry out trial therapy or purchase a device, the clinician, individual and carers must consider factors such as:
  - ◆ Does the device comes with a warranty?
  - ◆ How long does the warranty lasts?
  - ◆ How much will it cost to insure the device?
  - ◆ What are the service policies of the company who supply the device?

At this stage we often advise the individual, other professionals and carers to contact individuals who already have the particular communication aid. It is best policy that individuals gather as much knowledge about the particular device as possible, and very often other users can give them different perspectives from the clinician on using a communication aid, and using a specific communication aid.

Vanderheiden & Lloyd (1983) identify criteria which should be met when considering whether a communication system is functional for the individual. These are:

- The system must be useful for all communication functions and tasks.
- It must allow the user to interact with all communication partners and in all environments.
- It must allow for efficient and effective communication and maximise conversational control.
- It must allow for individual development, that is, for increasingly complex messages.

- It must be easily integrated into the individual's social and physical environments.
- It must interface with current systems – for example, seating, environmental controls, etc.
- It must be purchased without financial hardship.

Summary Sheets
- The clinician can use the summary sheets as an aid to evaluating use of the device.
- The VOCA Summary Sheet (Sample Form 13) has an open format to facilitate the individuality of the person being assessed.
- The VOCA Summary Checklist (Sample Form 14) is a means of coordinating the information obtained.

VOCA Summary Sheet

Name _____ **Date** _____

VOCA trialled	Positive features	Negative features	Summary of suitability
1			
2			
3			
4			
5			
6			

Signed _____

Sample Form 13 *VOCA summary sheet*

VOCA Summary Checklist

Name _____ **Date** _____

CLINICIAN'S RECOMMENDATIONS

NAME OF CLINICIAN _____

The communication aid should be ☐ static ☐ dynamic

The communication aid should be ☐ dedicated ☐ integrated

Access should be ☐ direct ☐ via switches ☐ no. of switches

The communication aid should be ☐ portable ☐ mounted

Other considerations _____

_____

_____

_____

Clinician's specific recommendation _____

The communication aid should be ☐ rented ☐ purchased

USER'S/CARER'S COMMENTS

NAME OF USE: _____

NAME OF CARER/S _____

Do the user/carers want to proceed with an AAC system? ☐ YES ☐ NO

If no, why not? _____

If yes, what is the specific preference? _____

_____

_____

Reasons for preference _____

_____

_____

Sample Form 14 *VOCA summary checklist*

LOCAL SERVICE PROVIDER COMMENTS

NAME OF LOCAL SERVICE PROVIDER _____

If there is a specific preference, for which device and why? _____

_____

_____

Are there specific issues which need to be addressed? _____

_____

_____

_____

NEEDS

Identify needs during diagnostic/initial period _____

_____

_____

Who will be responsible for fulfilling these needs _____

_____

_____

FUNDING

How will the device be funded? _____

_____

Who will pursue this? _____

_____

REVIEW

Date/Time frame _____

Signed _____

Sample Form 14 *Continued*

CHAPTER 17

The Partially Verbal Individual: Special Considerations

Introduction

There is one issue that requires special consideration in the process of AAC prescription, and there is no easy answer to the problem it presents. This is the individual who is deemed sufficiently unintelligible by the clinician to warrant AAC implementation, but who does not want augmentation or 'replacement' of his speech through either low or high technology. Competence in intelligibility is usually a judgement call, and this is reflected nowhere as much as in this particular area where the opinion of the clinician and the potential user or carers conflict.

The Characteristics of the Individual

Although no specific characteristics apply to this group and individual factors must always be considered, there may be a number of features that are applicable.

- Their experience with any alternative means of communication may have been limited.
- Communication therapy to improve intelligibility may have met with limited success.
- Communication needs may not be large.

- Their experience of communication with an extended range of partners and in a variety of non-aided situations may be limited. They have a restricted communication partner base which is usually reserved to carers and siblings. Their experience of communication in these settings and with these individuals, though still more limited than for normally developing individuals, is sufficiently successful.
- They tend to be relatively silent individuals, whose productions are limited in length – for example, single-word utterances – or non-existent. They tend not to extend themselves communicatively.
- They tend not to be initiators or generally spontaneous communicators with unfamiliar communication partners. If they are, this spontaneity is limited to familiar partners particularly, and familiar environments.
- They are aware of their limited intelligibility only to a certain point. Their tendency to limit their partner options, and their use of speech generally, have served to reduce the development of insight into their disability.
- They are extremely aware of their unintelligibility and this results in their reluctance to communicate or attempt change. These individuals typically refuse communication aids because the use of an aid would 'announce' their disability. They may feel they can hide behind silence. This inability to see a communication aid as beneficial to their independence extends usually to other pieces of equipment such as walkers or wheelchairs. Many individuals on the cusp of this category readily choose portable devices perhaps for this reason.
- They may not use cues or strategies readily to facilitate interpretation. They may be reminded to use contextual cues by their familiar partners.

The Characteristics of the Carer
Once again although individual differences between carers must always be kept in mind, there are a number of common features.

Their main or familiar communication partners may use strategies to facilitate intelligibility. These include:

- Phonemic cues, such as initial letter production. For example, 'Say the first letter';

- Semantic cues, such as 'Tell me what its like', 'Is it food?'
- Non-verbal cues such as pointing, facial expressions.
- A combination of cue types.

The main communication partners are usually one of two types:

1   *Over-interpreters and habitual facilitators of intelligibility* who use strategies to enhance communicative competence in the individual. They tend to anticipate routines and speech production, perhaps subconsciously. They are perhaps over-confident of their ability to interpret the individual's communications. When probes are used through barrier game strategies, they are surprised at the limitations of their interpreting skills (even if they are better than non-familiar communication partners) and the degree of the individual's unintelligibility. Habitual patterns have developed to compensate for intelligibility problems.

    One carer Berkery (1999), exemplifies beautifully the type of interaction that can develop.

Unless he is prodded, Ian reverts to being a regular Father Jack throwing out single words while the rest of the family try to guess exactly what he wants. The trouble is that in the family environment this system can work quite well and one word like "television" will produce the response "Do you want the television on?" "Do you want the station changed?"...The whole family participates in this shorthand almost unwittingly and the limitations of his speech only show up when he is in the day centre or hospital.

---

2   *Continual pressurisers* who request unobtainable accuracy of productions and frequent repetitions of utterance. Typically, these partners are unaware of the physical effort involved in speech production for the individual, and the impossibility of improving production by these means. These may be carers of individuals who have had a history of therapeutic input on speech production without success. (This raises the issues of more rapid diagnostic and decision-making skills for potentially non-verbal or partially verbal individuals.)

Defining Communicative Competence

When the demonstration and trialling of communication aids, low- or high-tech has been completed, and the carer and potential user are asked their opinions about proceeding, it may be at this point that issues of communicative competence really emerge. In this scenario, communication competence is usually defined by the judgement of intelligibility. Although standardised tools can be used to probe articulatory and phonological skills and oral motor function, judgement of intelligibility involves more than this. It is usually subjective and can vary between communication partners and environments. Because intelligibility is subjective, the judgement of it by carers and individuals is important and appropriate under these circumstances.

If differences exist between the clinician and the carers/indivduals, the clinician can be placed in somewhat of an ethical dilemma. Does she pursue her normal objective of communicative competence as she defines it, that is, the provision of an AAC system? Does she do her utmost to convince the carers and individual of the validity of this route? Or does she accept without question the carer's and individual's judgement of communicative competence? There really is no easy answer but to help in the decision making, the tools outlined in the following sections may be used.

Judgement of Intelligibility

Judgement of intelligibility is usually seen as having five dimensions:

1 Intelligibility by familiar or main communication partners
2 Intelligibility by unfamiliar communication partners
3 Intelligibility in familiar contexts/situations
4 Intelligibility in unfamiliar contexts/situations
5 Intelligibility in single and multi-word utterances.

A sixth judgement stage is proposed: that of

6 Self-judgement of intelligibility by the potential user.

The Tools

The following tools or types of tools may be used:

- Standardised assessment or informal probes of articulation, phonological skills and oral motor function.
- Judgement of Intelligibility by Communication Partners Rating Scale.
- Analysis of Communication Breakdown and Success.
- Video and Audio Analysis of Intelligibility.
- Auditory analysis of intelligibility via tools such as Dowden's (1997) Index of Augmented Speech Comprehensibility in Children (I-ASCC).

The use of normed or informal probes of articulatory and phonological skills will not be discussed here, as they are a standard part of all speech & language therapists' clinical repertoire.

Judgement of Intelligibility by Communication Partners Rating Scale
It is important to elicit judgements of the communication partner and the clinician during the AAC process. To achieve this, it is possible to use a rating scale (see Sample Form 15), which will facilitate understanding of and comparison of the judgements being made. This scale can be used with any relevant individuals. We recommend:

- The individual if appropriate
- The main carer/s
- The clinician assessing, and
- Local service providers – for example, educators.

A master copy can then be made to chart all communication partners' ratings. It may be best to colour code each participant's answers on the master copy. The scale can highlight the differences between familiar and unfamiliar partners. This helps to determine if intelligibility is an issue, and for whom. It also serves to identify environments, which may in some way influence intelligibility.

The rating can then be used to feed back to the individual and carers to inform them and to help develop insight into speech intelligibility. It can also be used to record changes in ratings over a

Judgement of Intelligibility Scale

Name of individual
Name of person filling in form
Relationship to individual
Date completed

1   How easy is it for you to understand _____'s speech? Please
     tick one of the following answers.

     No problem, always understand   [ ]

     Mostly easy, the odd time difficult   [ ]

     Sometimes difficult, sometimes OK   [ ]

     Mostly difficult, the odd time OK   [ ]

     Extremely difficult, rarely understand   [ ]

2   How would you rate _____'s speech intelligibility? Please tick
     one of the following answers.

     Very poor   [ ]

     Poor   [ ]

     OK   [ ]

     Good   [ ]

     Excellent   [ ]

Are there factors, which influence how well you understand _____'s
speech? Please tick one of the answers to each question.

3   When short sentences or single words are used, does this make a difference?

     Much easier to understand   [ ]

     A little bit easier to understand   [ ]

     Makes no difference   [ ]

     Makes it harder to understand   [ ]

Sample Form 15 *Judgement of intelligibility scale*

4 When non-verbal signals, such as pointing or facial expression, are used, does this makes a difference?

Much easier to understand

A little bit easier to understand

Makes no difference

Makes it harder to understand

5 When you understand the context – for example, talking about something you know, or something occurring at that moment does this makes a difference?

Much easier to understand

A little bit easier to understand

Makes no difference

Makes it harder to understand

6 When _____ repeats the word or sentence you have not understood, does this make a difference?

Much easier to understand

A little bit easier to understand

Makes no difference

Makes it harder to understand

7 When you use strategies to help _____'s intelligibility, does this make a difference?

Much easier to understand

A little bit easier to understand

Makes no difference

Makes it harder to understand

Sample Form 15 *Continued*

8 Can you give examples of:

Strategies you use that help   _____

Strategies you use that do not help   _____

Strategies _____ uses that help   _____

Strategies _____ uses that do not help   _____

Please comment on _____'s intelligibility in various situations. Please tick one of the answers to each question.

9 How is intelligibility at home?

Excellent   ☐

Good   ☐

OK   ☐

Poor   ☐

Very Poor   ☐

10 How is intelligibility in school/centre?

Excellent   ☐

Good   ☐

OK   ☐

Poor   ☐

Very Poor   ☐

11 How is intelligibility when talking to strangers?

Excellent   ☐

Good   ☐

OK   ☐

Poor   ☐

Very Poor   ☐

Sample Form 15 *Continued*

12 How is intelligibility in infrequent situations (identify) _____

Excellent ☐

Good ☐

OK ☐

Poor ☐

Very Poor ☐

13 Are there other factors that might influence _____'s
intelligibility? Please identify.

14 In overall terms, rate how happy you are with _____'s speech?

Very happy ☐

Happy ☐

Accepting ☐

Unhappy ☐

Very unhappy ☐

Sample Form 15 *Continued*

period of time, perhaps to help evaluate if the potential user is more 'ready' for AAC implementation.

Subsequent to completing the scales, the clinician can also make comparative lists to include information such as:

- Who rates the speaker as most intelligible?
- Who rates the speaker as least intelligible?
- Are ratings consistent among communication partners?

Analysis of Communication Breakdown and Success
The clinician can further judge the validity of the ratings achieved through the Judgement of Intelligibility Scale and increase the validity of analysis of the individual's intelligibility by evaluation of communication breakdowns and success in a familiar environment. This can be at home or school, or preferably in a number of familiar environments. If resource constraints are not a factor, then analysis in unfamiliar environments/contexts is a good idea. The comparison between performance in familiar and unfamiliar environments may help the individual and carers to understand the issue of intelligibility outside the home environment.

The easiest way to carry out this analysis is to use observer recording. Use of video recording and analysis through this medium is feasible, but use of video may impact on either communication partner's performance sufficiently to give a false picture. Minimal intrusion should be the rule. Therefore, the ideal observers are people already in that environment, such as a class teacher.

A simple chart, such as that in Sample Form 16, is best. Over-analysis may result from too much information. The main information required from this analysis is whether communication breakdowns result, and whether this is from the individual's speech intelligibility. However, the clinician may be able to filter out valuable information regarding factors such as interaction strategies. For example, in the sample in Table 17.1 it may be that non-directed choices give the individual a greater chance of success. We also find out that the individual is a child who initiates, and may benefit from modelling of speech as in example B.

Communication Success and Breakdown Recording Sheet

Name of individual ....

Name of observer ....

Date ....

Situation ....

Please chart the exact sequence of communication between the individual and the person with whom he/she is interacting. Use numbers (1, 2, 3, etc) to identify who is communicating and what they are saying. A number of interactions should be noted in this way. Identify a new interaction by underlining the previous one.

Communication sequence	Was the interaction a success or breakdown?	What (if any) cues or strategies did the individual use to get his message across?	What (if any) cues or strategies did the partner use to get his message across?

Sample Form 16 *Communication success and breakdown recording sheet*

Table 17.1 *Sample communication success and breakdown recording sheet*

Communication sequence	Was the interaction a success or breakdown?	What (if any) cues or strategies did the individual use to get his message across?	What (if any) cues or strategies did the partner use to get his message across?
Example A			
1 David: ?????? (UNINTELLIGIBLE)	Breakdown	Nil	Object selection
2 Teacher: What?			
3 David: ????? (UNINTELLIGIBLE)			
4 Teacher: Do you want the ball?			
5 David: *walks away*			
Example B			
1 Teacher: Hello	Success	Nodding head for yes	Non-directed choices
2 David: Ho			
3 Teacher: Do you want to play David?		Reaching for desired object	Simple language
4 David: Pay			
5 Teacher: Which one do you want, a ball or a book?			
6 David: Ba			
Example C			
1 David: Ball	Success – David achieved his goal.	Pointing	Nil
2 Teacher: Here you are.			

If you are asking another observer to fill in the form, give examples so that the information the clinician wants is in fact obtained. An example of this information is given.

Video and Audio Analysis of Intelligibility
Video or audio recording of the individual in a number of situations can facilitate in judgement of intelligibility. Examples include:
- Conversation with familiar partner (50–100 words)
- Conversation with unfamiliar partner (50–100 words)
- Picture description task (50–100 words)
- Single word naming task (25–50 words)

- A five-minute recording of each task is usually sufficient with further time allocated as necessary.
- Conversations in some cases may need to be facilitated. For example, the familiar partner may be advised to choose a topic concerning a recent event such as a family wedding, or a subject close to the individual's heart, such as football.
- Both communication partners (familiar and unfamiliar) should be advised to avoid adopting a dominant, questioning style in the interaction. Open questions such as 'Tell me about ...' may facilitate conversation best.
- The picture description task and single word naming task should involve stimuli that are not visible to the familiar partner. There is no real need to record the stimuli, as the issue revolves around whether the partners can understand the speech of the individual.
- The communication partners and clinician should transcribe and then analyse these tasks, and develop a judgement of intelligibility based on them. Differences between familiar and non-familiar partner may be identified, in addition to differences between sequenced and isolated speech productions. The familiar partner may also develop insight into the amount of communications made by the individual, the possible dominance of communications by one partner, and insight into issues around intelligibility not previously understood.
- A simple chart such as that shown in Sample Form 17 is sufficient for recording this information.

Analysis of Intelligibility by Task

Name of individual _____

Name of observer _____

Description of task _____

Date _____

Please write what you hear. If two people are talking together, write down what each person says, and in the order they say it.

Sample Form 17 *Analysis of intelligibility by task*

Index of Augmented Speech Comprehensibility in Children (I-ASCC)
Dowden (1997) uses a measure that evaluates factors that impact on speech comprehensibility, that is, issues discussed thus far regarding partner familiarity and semantic content. She states that this measure facilitates decision making. It helps to:

• Resolve team conflicts regarding speech versus augmentation
• Demonstrate the benefit of speech supplementation strategies, and
• Demonstrate the limitation of speech supplementation for children who require augmentation.

Dowden's measure, which can be used clinically, is based on published lists of selected vocabulary for children from birth to seven years. Potential users are tape-recorded saying the word list. Familiar and unfamiliar partners transcribe the utterance under two conditions:

1   Audio only (that is, no context), and
2   Audio with written cue (semantic context condition).

Dowden's example of a written cue is as follows:

'Something children eat for a snack.'

The target word in this case is 'cracker'. Dowden's tool is a valid instrument for pursuing the objectives she has outlined.

Where to From Here?
The results from these instruments can be used to help determine which path to proceed on. These options include:

• Drop AAC as an alternative.
• Consider strategies for improving the intelligibility of speech.
• Use the information obtained from the above tools to develop insight.
• Determine whether to review the situation after a period of time when independence of thought and action may be more valued, or needs changed.

- Consider partial augmentation – for example, a low-tech system or small portable device for certain situations.
- Consider a period of trial on a device to further address the question of the appropriateness of an AAC system.

The clinician has no right to prescribe without considering the factors outlined above in cases where the individual or carer of a partially verbal individual does not see the benefit of using a communication system. No one will receive any benefits when a system is implemented without due consideration of the needs and attitudes of the users and carers. Everything possible needs to be done in order to determine the validity of the prescription process and to accurately match the system with the individual it is being prescribed for. The clinician's job is to facilitate the user and carers to make an informed decision, even if this decision is to reject augmentation as a possibility.

CHAPTER 18

The Diagnostic Period

The diagnostic period does not only apply to high-tech systems. It can just as easily apply to low-tech systems such as communication boards. When implementing any new system, the clinician should regularly review it, in order to ensure that it meets the needs of the individual, and that it develops along with the individual.

With regard to high-tech systems, when the initial phase of the assessment process is complete and the next phase begins, the clinician should provide the user with specific information and guidelines for ensuring the communication aid is given a proper trial. This may include specific details on, for example:

- How to programme the aid and add in new information
- How to charge the aid
- Where the switch point is and how to place switches
- How the aid should be mounted
- What situations it should be used in
- Contact numbers for clinician and manufacturers in case problems arise.

The clinician may find it advisable to make at least one domiciliary visit during the diagnostic period to facilitate use of the communication aid and problem solving.

Prior to attending the review appointment the following should be sent to the carers and service providers:

- The AAC review appointment sheet (Sample Form 18) to remind the individual, carer and others of the appointment date.
- The AAC trial summary sheet (Sample Form 19) to help the clinician address issues effectively and assess outcome. This should ideally be filled in by the individual, if appropriate, the carer and the service providers.

During the review session, the clinician needs to:

- Observe the individual using the system
- Identify problem areas
- Identify positive developments
- Elicit user, carer and local professional opinion about the system and its suitability for the individual as measured by them
- Identify the way forward.

A second period of diagnostic therapy may be advisable in some cases.

Individuals with physical disability may require a number of ongoing assessments and re-evaluation for some or all of the following:

- The individual's postural changes and sitting position while using the switch
- The functional seating system
- The placement and functional use of the switch
- The type of mounting system for the switch
- The method and/or speed of scanning on the device.

With close monitoring, the individual should be improving in the skills of switch use, scanning and communication system use.

Augmentative and Alternative Communication Review

Date

To

Address

Re

DOB

Address

Dear

As you know, the review date for the above named has been arranged for:

Day

Date

Time

We would be grateful if, prior to attendance, you would fill in the enclosed summary sheet to help us in planning the session. Please post it to reach us before the review date along with your confirmation that you will be attending.

Yours sincerely

Speech & Language Therapy Department

Sample Form 18 *Augmentative and alternative communication review appointment letter*

Augmentative and Alternative Communication Trial Summary

Name of user _____

Period of trial _____

Name of system _____

Please answer the following questions.

1 Was the system used by the user? Please identify how often, by ticking one of the boxes below:

☐ Never ☐ Seldom ☐ Sometimes ☐ Often ☐ Always

2 Did the user have difficulties in using the system?

☐ Yes ☐ No

If so, please identify these difficulties. Please be as specific as possible.

_____

_____

_____

_____

3 How did the user feel about the system generally? Please comment by ticking one of the boxes below and adding any additional information.

☐ Hated ☐ Disliked ☐ No obvious reaction ☐ Liked ☐ Loved

_____

_____

_____

_____

Sample Form 19 *Augmentative and alternative communication trial summary sheet*

4   Did the user actually get to use the system?

☐ Yes   ☐ No

If so, please identify in what situations and how often. If not, please identify in what situations he was not able to use it in and why.

Situation in which aid was used	How often?	Why do you think it was used in this situation?

Situation in which aid was not used	How often?	Why do you think it was not used in this situation?

5   What do you feel the positive features of the system were?

(a) ....

(b) ....

(c) ....

(d) ....

Sample Form 19 *Continued*

6 What do you feel the negative features of the system were?

(a) _____

(b) _____

(c) _____

(d) _____

7 If the system did not meet all the user's needs, what do we need to do to improve this?

Need not met	Why not?	How can we improve on this?

8 Is an augmentative communication system generally appropriate for this individual?

☐ Yes ☐ No

Why? _____

9 Is this communication system an appropriate route for this individual?

☐ Yes ☐ No

Why? _____

10 Other comments

_____

_____

_____

Signed _____ **Date** _____

Sample Form 19 *Continued*

CHAPTER 19

Final Points

> The ultimate goal of AAC intervention is not to find a technical
> solution to the communication problem, but to enable the individual
> to efficiently and effectively engage in a variety of interactions.
>
> *Beukelman & Mirenda (1992, p7)*

Protocol

Many individuals are referred for assessment of augmentative
communication potential. Some of these individuals will not be
candidates for an AAC system. The aim of assessment is to:

- Exclude those who are not suitable candidates (for whatever reason)
- Identify through detailed assessment those who are candidates for AAC
- Identify what the options are for these individuals.

AAC prescription should follow guidelines. The following are
recommended although both the sequence and the validity of conducting
each section should be determined by the clinician.

1 Referral
2 Appointment information and further identification information
   including reason for referral

3　Observation of the individual in communication environments

4　Assessment of early AAC skills or multi-sensory stimuli, if appropriate

5　Assessment of language and literacy skills

6　Assessment of symbolic skills

7　Assessment of access

8　Assessment of scanning

9　Assessment on voice-output communication aids

10　Summary observations

11　Diagnostic therapy

12　Review

13　Prescription.

Summary Questions

Summary questions will help the clinician and others in understanding how to move forward and apply all the information learned during the assessment process. The intention is to identify user needs and match the technology available to these needs. They should include the following:

- What is the individual's and carer's motivation for using an AAC system?
- Would an AAC system be motivating for the individual and his communication partners?
- What are the individual's communication needs? Does an AAC system need to provide the full range of communication functions?
- Is the individual communicating satisfactorily currently, according to individual, carer, local service provider and the clinician?
- Based on observations and analysis of skills and other issues is an AAC system appropriate for this individual?
- Is there a particular area of difficulty that needs to be addressed before proceeding with an AAC system?
- Should this system be low-tech or high-tech or both?
- Would an AAC system enhance and facilitate communication development?
- Would an AAC system be harmonious with other issues in the individual's life and promote interaction with communication partners?

- What are the specific features of the system needed?
- Is it likely that the individual's communication needs will change over time and what impact will this have on an AAC system?
- Should the AAC system be integrated or dedicated, if it is high-tech?
- What is the individual's preference?
- Are there support systems present for the implementation of the AAC system in the carer's immediate environment?
- If the system is high tech, is there support from the company in the form of manuals, warranties and service?
- Is an AAC system affordable?
- Which is the better option, diagnostic therapy or immediate prescription?

In general, we feel the most important questions to ask centre around the motivation and user preference. These in themselves will frequently help to determine the way forward.

Funding

We must of course mention funding. As referred to previously, our policy is not to consider the funding issue until we have made a decision with the user, carers and local service providers about prescription, as it is not a clinical issue. Our primary goal is to evaluate the potential of the individual for augmentative and alternative communication. However, the clinician must consider all the variables related to augmentative and alternative communication, and the benefits of providing AAC for an individual can be greatly impacted upon if potential problems such as funding are not addressed.

Funding can be problematic to discuss in general terms as funding practices vary greatly from service to service, and the clinician will have to take into account how funding is practised locally. If there are particular problems, as Church & Glennen (1992, p22) state:

Resourceful professionals who are willing to seek out all possible funding sources can almost always find money.

The general means of funding are:

- Area Health Authorities
- Private resources, and
- Voluntary groups.

Yorkston & Karlan (1992) have identified four levels of need which relate to the selection of communication aids. These can also be applied to funding of communication aids when making a case for funding and these are:

1 Needs are currently met, that is, the individual has a satisfactory means of communicating
2 Mandatory, that is, essential
3 Desirable, that is, important but not essential
4 Unimportant, that is, not considered.

It must be noted, however, that when considering funding, the clinician should bear in mind that communication is a right, not an option, for disabled individuals.

Information Sharing

An important part of augmentative communication is sharing information with the users, carers and professionals. Why?
- This is not only their right, but essential to ensuring the successful implementation of AAC systems.
- It includes them as partners in the prescription process.
- It provides them with realistic options – for example, an understanding that AAC is not a miracle cure, and that it is not a natural system which communication partners in their environments will readily understand.
- It prepares them for their role in AAC implementation.
- It addresses concerns, such as reinforcing that AAC is not a replacement of the individual's communication modes and that it does not inhibit vocal development.
- It ensures they are responsible for AAC prescription and implementation.

Extended Evaluation

Church & Glennen (1992) describe AAC assessment as 'extended evaluation'. This is the nature of prescription in AAC. It is not a one-off process. It is time consuming for all those concerned.

1   The assessment period itself can be lengthy as it involves evaluation of multiple components which can interact with each other to make assessment difficult. This is especially true for individuals who are physically disabled to a severe degree.
2   The decision-making process can be lengthy and involve periods of waiting while particular issues such as seating are problem solved.
3   The diagnostic period is an additional time component, which, while not essential for all individuals, can be vital for others.
4   It is not the prescription process itself which can be lengthy. Once a person adopts AAC, there can be a lifetime commitment by service providers to supporting the user and others and to reviewing needs.

What this of course means is that the cost of AAC assessment (and therapy) in terms of both time and money can be significant, particularly for individuals who present with severe disabilities. However, there is no doubt to clinicians who see the benefits, that these costs are vindicated. One only has to look at the outcomes in terms of communication, interaction and independence which result from AAC.

Summary Note

Augmentative and alternative communication is powerless unless it is appropriately and accurately prescribed and unless it is implemented correctly. It can only be successful if the skills the user brings to AAC, as well as the problems which need to be addressed, are properly understood, harnessed and remedied. It involves knowledge of both communication and technology on the part of all concerned. However, it is not about technology specifically. AAC is about the user. It is about empowering the individual.

Appendix

Introduction of Product Examples

This list is not intended to be exhaustive and clinicians should contact companies for specific details of their products.

For AAC devices, Rumble & Larcher's (1998) *AAC Device Review* provides a comprehensive review.

The reader's attention is drawn to the European Communities (Medical Devices) Regulations Directive 93/42/EEC concerning general medical devices (MDD).

Technical equipment is subject to obsolescence and the following details are current at time of writing only.

Low-Tech Systems

Company	Product Names	Product Type
Winslow Press Telford Road Bicester Oxon OX26 4LQ UK	Colour communication stickers	Pick 'n Stick packs. Also on IBM compatible disk and CD-Rom
	Pocket Holders	77 x 115mm (3 x 5 inch) small portable folders. Clear vinyl pockets
	Communication boards	Plastic. Waterproof. Carry handle. Two sizes
	Eye-Com board	Eye pointing system. Transparent. Acrylic. Wooden stand

Low-Tech Systems *continued*

Company	Product Names	Product Type
Winslow Press *continued*	Communication notebooks	Small. Portable. Looseleaf. Blank sheets. Colour-coded dividers
	Picture Communication Symbols (PCS)	Books 1, 2 and 3 etc. Containing symbols
	Boardmaker	Software programme for producing more than 3,000 colour symbols. PCS symbols. Variety of languages. Drawing programme. Pre-made grids. Text and non-text options
	Communication folders, wallets and books	Various
	Makaton database (core vocabulary and National Curriculum)	IBM compatible graphics files for all Makaton signs and symbols
	Writing with Symbols 2000	Word and symbol processor
	Clicker 4	Communication & writing tool
Cambridge Adaptive The Mount Toft Cambridge CB3 7RL UK	Rotary Indicator	Magnetic surface with lever switch (other switches optional). Can be used with magnetic materials, drawings or objects
IRISH AGENT Codicom Ltd Corville Roscrea, Co. Tipperary	E-Tran Frame	Perspex transparent frame which can be used with symbols, words, pictures or objects. Wheel base, weighted base or clamp base
Imaginart Inc 307 Arizona Street Bisbee AZ 85603 USA	Colour communication stickers	Pick 'n Stick packs. Also on IBM compatible disk and CD-ROM
	Communication boards	As above
	Eye-Com board	As above
Mayer Johnson PO Box 1579 Solona Beach CA 92075-7579 USA	Boardmaker	As above
	Picture Communication Symbols	As above
	Communication folders, wallets and books	Various

Low-Tech Systems *continued*

Company	Product Names	Product Type
Incredible Design Company Chailey Heritage Enterprise Centre Chailey Heritage North Chailey Near Lewes East Sussex BN8 4EF UK	Chailey Communication System	Communication system which grows with the developing child. Designed to incorporate any alternative system or combination of systems (eg, pictures, Rebus, Bliss, etc)
Access First PO Box 3990 Glen Allen VA 23058-3990 USA	Comboard	Battery driven dial scanner for selecting from a choice of pictures/symbols. Switch access.
Easiaids Ltd 5 Woodcote Park Avenue Purley Surrey CR8 3NH UK	Rotary Indicator	As previously

Voice-Output Communication Aids

Company	Product Names	Product Type
Access First PO Box 3990 Glen Allen VA 23058-3990 USA	Ultimate Ultimate 8	Static. Digitised. 4 location. Each location at 4 seconds each. Portable. Direct access. As above. 8 location at 4 seconds each. Direct and indirect access.
Cambridge Adaptive The Mount Toft Cambridge CB3 7RL UK *IRISH AGENT* Codicom Ltd Corville Roscrea Co. Tipperary	Cameleon Cameleon Express	Dynamic computer with Words + software. Symbols and text-based (EZ Keys) software packages available. Variable location (up to 128). Synthetic speech. Direct (touch screen optional) and indirect (switches, mouse, headpointer) access. Auditory scanning As above. Portable

Voice-Output Communication Aids *continued*

Company	Product Names	Product Type
Cambridge Adaptive *continued*	**Software** Talking Screens	PCS (Picture Communication Symbols) or nearly 2,500 Bliss symbols
	EZ Keys	Literacy based. Over 2,000 root words in dictionary. Word prediction
	Chailey Communication System	Over 3,500 Rebus symbols (black and white) organised by topic around the needs of the National Curriculum
	Ingfield Dynamic Vocabularies	Over 2,500 PCS symbols at four levels which increase in cognitive demand and communication potential
	Message Mate	Static. Portable. 1/2/4/5/10/20/40/ locations. Four levels. Digitised speech. Direct and indirect access. Auditory scanning (word)
	Mini Message Mate	As above. 8 location only
Common Cents Systems PO Box 1180 Litchfield CT 06759 USA	Box Talk	Static. Portable. Digitised speech. Direct and indirect access. 9/16 location
Easiaids Ltd 5 Woodcote Park Avenue Purley Surrey CR8 3NH UK	Lightwriter/ Macaw/QED Memowriter/Zygo Parrot/Fourtalk/ Spokesman/Portacom	See below
	PAC 6/10	Static. Indirect access. 6 /10 location. Optional interface for BBC computer
	Digimax	Static. Portable. Digitised speech. 2/3/8/12/32/48 locations. Eight to 48 levels. LCD display
Frame Technologies W681 Pearl Street Oneida WI 54155 USA	Voice-in-a-Box	Static. Portable. Direct and indirect (4 messages) access. Digitised speech. 16 location
	Voice-in-a-Box/ 6 level	As above with up to six levels of messages

Voice-Output Communication Aids *continued*

Company	Product Names	Product Type
Frame Technologies *continued*	MicroVoice/16	Static. Portable. 16 location. Direct access
	TalkPad	Static. Portable. Rugged. Carry handle. 4 location
Franklin 7 Windmill Business Village Brooklands Close Sunbury Middlesex TW16 7DY UK *IRISH AGENT* Addex Limited Three Rock Road Sandyford Dublin 18.	Language Master	Dynamic screen. Special Edition Language Master (LM600SE) . Literacy based. Over 300,000 definitions. Over 500,000 synonyms and antonyms. Grammar guide. Audible pronunciations. Stores personal messages. User customisation for variety of special needs
Liberator Ltd Whitegates Swinstead Lincolnshire NG33 4PA UK	Alphatalker	Static. Portable. Single icon and semantic compaction. Minspeak. Digitised speech. 4/8/32 location. Direct and indirect access. Themes. Auditory scanning (word). Icon prediction
	Deltatalker	Static. Portable. Single icon and semantic compaction. Minspeak. Digitised and synthetic speech. 8/32/128 location. Environmental controls. PC connection. Direct and indirect (switches, headpointer, etc) access. Auditory scanning. Icon prediction. LCD display
	ChatBox (CB2)	Static. Portable. 16 locations. Four levels. Minspeak icons (or other symbols). Direct and indirect access. Icon prediction
	Chatbox DX	As above plus auditory prompts, 4 location overlays, additional switch jacks to operate the locations individually
	Walker Talker	Static aid. Portable. Digitised speech. 16 locations. Direct access

Voice-Output Communication Aids *continued*

Company	Product Names	Product Type
Liberator *continued*	Vanguard	Dynamic with Minspeak. 4/8/45 location. Digitised and synthetic speech. Direct and indirect (including headpointer) access. Auditory scanning. Icon prediction. Environmental controls and computer connection. Large text option. Word prediction option
	Axs 1600	Portable. Computer with Windows software. Dynamic with text-based and symbol-based software options. Text-based package includes word prediction and abbreviation expansion. Touchscreen. Direct and indirect access
	Liberator	Static. 8/32/128 locations. Minspeak. Synthetic speech. Direct and indirect access. Auditory scanning. Icon prediction. LCD display
	Bigmack	Single-channel voice-output switch
	One Step	Static. Portable. Digitised speech. Single message. A number can connect together
	Speakeasy	Static. Portable. Digitised. 12 locations. Direct and indirect access (via 12 individual switches)
	Step by step	Static. Portable. Digitised speech. Can store up to 45 messages in sequence. Number of switch hits corresponds to the message number.
	Sidekick	Portable. Static. 24 location. Direct and indirect access. Icon prediction. Auditory prompts.
	Software	
	Language Living and Learning	For Deltatalker, Vanguard and Liberator. 128 location. Up to 5,000 words and sentences. Predominately two with some three hit activations

Voice-Output Communication Aids *continued*

Company	Product Names	Product Type
Liberator *continued*	Unity A/T	For Alphatalker. Compact version of Unity
	Word Strategy	For Deltatalker and Liberator. 128 location. Over 4,000 words. Two and three hit activations
	Unity	For Deltatalker (128 version), Vanguard (for Vanguard) and Liberator (for Liberator). Up to 5,000 words and sentences. Two and three hit activations
	Stepping Stones	For Alphatalker, Liberator and Deltatalker. Based on LLL. Over 750 words. 32 locations. Predominantly two hit activations
	Unity Condensed	For Liberator and Deltatalker. Over 3,000 words. Two hit activation
	Unichat 16	MiniMAP for Chatbox. Bases on Unity. 16 location. 10 overlays
	Pathways to LLL	MiniMAP based on LLL. For individuals not yet able to cope with LLL. 128 location. One and two hit activations
	WiVik2 Scan and WiVik Software	Simple text-based communication package. On Axs 1600
Mardis Business Development Centre Fylde Avenue Lancaster University Lancaster LA1 4YR UK	Eclipse	Static. Portable. Digitised speech. Direct and indirect access (depends on model). 2/4/8/16/32/64/128 locations. 128 levels. Talking menu
	Orac	Static. Portable. Single icon and semantic compaction. Digitised and synthetic speech. LCD display. 2/4/8/16/32/64/128 locations. Direct and indirect (including headpointer) access. Icon prediction
	Software 8 is great!	For Eclipse. Introductory package. Various topics. 16 coloured overlays in 8 location

Voice-Output Communication Aids *continued*

Company	Product Names	Product Type
Mardis *continued*	Reach for the Stars	For Eclipse. Package moves from words to sentences. 128 overlay and two hit activation. Topic based. Fast recharge. Disc drive powered by Eclipse
	Talking Lifestyles	For Orac. 64/128 location. Mostly two hit activation
Mayer Johnson PO Box 1579 Solona Beach CA 92075-7579 USA	Hand Held Voice	Dynamic. Portable. Digitised speech. Black & white LCD. Direct access. 9 location. 32 pages. Expansion cards available
	Tech Four	4 messages. 4 overlay. 4 seconds per message. Battery operated. Water resistant. Portable. Digitised. Static. 6 colour overlays. Dual access
	Tech Talk	Static. 8 messages. 6/8/12 levels available with increasing memory per level.
	Tech Speak	Static. 32 messages. 2/4/6 level with increasing memory per level
	Software Speaking Dynamically Pro	Software speech output communication programme. Variety of access methods. Word prediction
	Touchscreens	Mount on monitors to make PC touch accessible. Magic touch made of glass. Edmark Touch made of plastic
Microtechnology Unit Sandwell EDC Popes Lane Oldbury B69 4PJ UK	Echo 4	Portable. Digitised speech. 4 locations. Indirect access
GB Ritchie 21 Whetstone Close Heelands Milton Keynes MK13 7PP UK	The Barry Box	Portable. Static. 48 location (also 64 location). Direct access

Voice-Output Communication Aids *continued*

Company	Product Names	Product Type
Sunrise Medical Ltd Sunrise Business Park High Street Wollaston West Midlands DY8 4PS UK	Dynavox	Dynamic. Some pre-programmed page sets. Dynasyms/PCS symbols. Synthetic speech. Direct (touch screen) and indirect access. Nearly 3,500 symbols. Pre-stored templates. 1-72 locations. Auditory scanning. Draw facility. Zoom facility. Song manager. Alarm system.
	Dynamite	As above. Portable. 1-54 locations
	Easy Talk	Static. Portable. 1/2/4/10/20/40 locations. Four levels. Digitised speech. Direct and indirect access. Auditory scanning (beep)
	Digivox	Static. Portable. Digitised speech. 2/3/8/12/32/48 locations. Eight to 48 levels. Direct and indirect access. Auditory scanning. Icon prediction. LCD display
	Dynamo	Black-and-white dynamic. Digitised speech. 30 minutes recording time. Direct and indirect access. Infra-red.
	Software Gateway	For Dynavox and Dynamite. 1,000 words for three- to twelve-year-olds
QED Ability House 242 Gosport Road Fareham Hampshire PO16 0SS UK	Macaw	Static. Portable. Single icon and semantic compaction. 2/4/8/16/32/128 locations. Thirty two levels. Direct and indirect access. Digitised speech. Auditory scanning
IRISH AGENT Codicom Limited Corville Roscrea Co. Tipperary	Portacom	Static. Portable. Single icon. Direct and indirect access. Digitised speech. 1/2/4/10/20/40 locations. Auditory scanning (beep). Alarm

Voice-Output Communication Aids *continued*

Company	Product Names	Product Type
QED *continued*	Fourtalk	Static. Direct and indirect access. 1/2/4 locations. Digitised speech. Portable
	Twintalk	As above, but twice the size
	Zygo Parrot	Static. Portable. Digitised speech. Direct or indirect (JK model) access. 16 location
	VoicePal	Up to five messages through Taction Pads connected to objects
	VoicePal Plus	Static. Up to 10 six-second messages. Direct and indirect access. Taction Pads as above
	DAVE	Static. Digitised speech. 4/16 locations. Indirect access
	Vocaid	Static. Portable. 35 locations. Range of overlays. Synthetic speech. Direct access. Bliss, Rebus. Colours. Optional amplifier
	Lightwriter	As for Toby Churchill
	QED Memowriter	Portable. Direct and indirect access. QWERTY layout. Sensitive keys. Built-in keyguard. Display and printer. Audio feedback
	Zygo Secretary	As above plus 20 recorded speech messages. Stores messages for retrieval later
	Cameleon	As for Cambridge Adaptive
Techcess Ltd Unit 12 Willow Park Industrial Estate Upton Lane Stoke Golding Nuneaton Warwickshire CV13 6EU UK	Blackhawk	Portable. Digitised speech. 16 locations. 4 levels. Direct access
	Hawk	Static. Portable. Digitised speech. 8 locations. 2 levels. Direct and indirect access (via 8 separate switches)
	Superhawk	Static. Digitised speech. 1/2/3/4/6/8/9/12/18/36/72 locations. 72 levels. Direct and indirect access. Auditory scanning. LCD display.

203

Voice-Output Communication Aids *continued*

Company	Product Names	Product Type
Toby Churchill Ltd 20 Panton Street Cambridge CB2 1HP UK *IRISH AGENT* Codicom Ltd Corville Roscrea Co. Tipperary	Lightwriter	Static. Portable. Literacy system. Synthetic speech. Various options including keyboard layout (ABC or QWERTY), display (LCD or VFD) etc. Direct (SL35) and indirect (SL85 model) access. Direct model has options of rubber or light touch keyboards. Dual display. Dectalk optional. Auditory prompts (SL35) or scanning (SL85). Word prediction. Synthetic speech. Foreign language synthesisers
	Spokesman	Static. Portable. 1/2/4/8/16 location. Digitised speech. Optional symbol book. Direct and indirect access.

Switches

Company	Product Names	Product Type
Liberator Ltd Whitegates Swinstead Lincolnshire NG33 4PA UK	**Able Net** **Single Switches** Big Red switch Jelly Bean switch Specs switch	 Large. Strong pressure Medium. Sensitive switches Small. Auditory/tactile feedback
	Accessories Jelly Bean Holder Switch Latch & Timer	 2/4 bean holder gives recessed effect to switches Allows latched and timed control
QED Ability House 242 Gosport Road Fareham Hampshire PO16 0SS UK	**Single Switches** QED Lever, Sub-miniature Lever Micro Lever switch QED adjustable pressure switch	 Pressure switches activated at one end. Auditory/tactile feedback Pressure Pad. Adjustable sensitivity. Head Pad. Squeeze ball

Switches *continued*

Company	Product Names	Product Type
IRISH AGENT	Tash Single switches	As above
Codicom Limited	Tash Double	As above
Corville	switches	
Roscrea	Tash Multiple	As above
Co. Tipperary	switches	
	Zygo Leaf switch	Two-way deflection switch
	Accessories	
	QED Multi-function latching box and timer	Allows latched and timed control of devices/toys
Techcess Ltd	**Tash single switches**	
Unit 12	Bubbles switch	Touch sensitive
Willow Park Industrial Estate	Untouchable Buddy	Adjustable pressure-sensitive switch. Auditory/tactile feedback
Stoke Golding	Buddy Button	Strong pressure-sensitive switch
Nuneaton	switches	Auditory/tactile feedback
Warwickshire CV13 6EU	Micro Light	Very light touch-sensitive switch
UK		Auditory/tactile feedback
	Leaf switch	Light pressure in one direction Auditory/tactile feedback
	Tip switch	Activated by tilting switch 5°
	Foot switch	Durable pressure switch Auditory/tactile feedback
	Cup/Mini cup switch	Small durable pressure switches Auditory/tactile feedback
	Tash Dual Switches	
	Rocker switch	Any part of top surface can activate. Auditory/tactile feedback
	Tash Multiple Switches	
	Wafer	5 membrane switches on one board
	Star	5 Recessed switches. Auditory/tactile feedback

Mounting Systems

Company	Product Names	Product Type
Liberator Ltd Whitegates Swinstead Lincolnshire NG33 4PA UK	Able Net Slim Armstrong Mounting System Able Net Universal Switch Mounting System	Very versatile assessment mounting system for switches Adjustable mounting system for switches
QED Ability House 242 Gosport Road Fareham Hampshire PO16 0SS UK *IRISH AGENT* Codicom Limited Corville Roscrea Co. Tipperary	Mobilia System 2000	Wide range of mounting systems for switches, communication aids, etc. Includes a 'Bendy Pole'
Techcess Ltd Unit 12 Willow Park Industrial Estate Stoke Golding Nuneaton CV13 6EU Warwickshire UK	DaeSSy Stem System DaeSSy Wheelchair Mounting System Device Holders/ Mounting Plates	Versatile, adjustable mounting system for switches Range of wheelchair mounts from foldable, to swing away for communication devices To attach communication devices/computers to mounting system

References

Baker B, 1985, 'The use of words and phrases on a Minspeak communication system', *Communication Outlook,* 7(1), pp8–10.

Berger AF, Presperin J & Tallman T, 1990, *'Positioning for Function',* *Wheelchairs and other Assistive Technology,* Valhalla Rehabilitation Publications Ltd, Valhalla, NY.

Berkery P, 1999 'Getting to Grips with New Technology: A parent's viewpoint', *ISAAC Ireland Newsletter*, June 1999.

Beukelman D & Mirenda P, 1992, *Augmentative and Alternative Communication: Management of Severe Communication Disorders in Children and Adults*, Paul Brookes Publishing, Baltimore.

Bzoch KR & League R, 1991, *Receptive–Expressive Emergent Language Test: A Method for Assessing the Language Skills of Infants*, 2nd Edition, Pro Ed, Austin, Texas.

Church G & Glennen S, 1992, *The Handbook of Assistive Technology,* Singular Publishing, San Diego, Ca.

Cook AM & Hussey SM, 1995, *Assistive Technologies: Principles and Practice*, Mosby, St Louis.

Coupe J, Barber M & Murphy D, 1988, 'Affective Communication', J Coupe & J Goldbart (eds), *Communication Before Speech: Normal Development and Impaired Communication,* Chapman and Hall, London.

Dewart H & Summers S, 1995, *The Pragmatics Profile of Everyday Communication Skills in Children*, NFER-Nelson, Windsor.

Dowden PA, 1997, 'Augmentative and Alternative Decision Making for Children with Severely Unintelligible Speech', *Augmentative and Alternative Communication*, 13, pp48–58.

Kent RD, Miolo G & Bloedell S, 1994, 'The Intelligibility of Children's Speech: A Review of Evaluation Procedures', *American Journal of Speech Language Pathology: A Journal of Clinical Practice*, 3, pp81–95.

Kiernan C & Reid B, 1987, *Pre-Verbal Communication Schedule*, NFER-Nelson, Windsor.

McCurtin A, 1994, 'A Preliminary Investigation into the use of Tests for Prelinguistic Assessment by Speech & Language Therapists.' Unpublished MSc Thesis. City University, London.

Musselwhite CR & St Louis K, 1988, *Communication Programming for Persons with Severe Handicaps: Vocal and Augmentative Strategies*, College Hill Press, Boston.

Reichle J, 1991, 'Defining the Decisions Involved in Designing and Implementing Augmentative and Alternative Communication Systems', J Reichle, J York & J Sigafoos (eds), *Implementing Augmentative and Alternative Communication: Strategies for Learners with Severe Disabilities*, Paul H Brookes Publishing Co, Baltimore, Ma.

Rumble G & Larcher J, 1998, *AAC Device Review*, Vocation, Marlow.

Shane HC, 1986, *Goals and Uses in Augmentative Communication: An Introduction*, Speech and Language Hearing Association, Rockville, Ma.

Smith MM, 1996, 'The Medium or the Message: A Study of Speaking Children Using Communication Boards', S von Tetzchner & M Hygun Jensen (eds), *Augmentative and Alternative Communication: European Perspectives*, Whurr Publishers, London.

Vanderheiden G & Lloyd L, 1983. 'Communication Systems and their Components', SW Blackstone & DM Bruskin (eds), *Augmentative Communication: An Introduction*, American Speech and Hearing Association, Rockville, Ma.

Wetherby AM & Prizant BM, 1993, *Communication and Symbolic Behaviour Scales*, Applied Symbolix, Chicago, Ill.

Yorkston KM & Karlan G, 1992, 'Assessment Procedures in Augmentative Communication: An Introduction', KM Yorkston (ed), *Augmentative Communication in the Medical Setting*, Communication Skill Builders, Tucson, Az.